Nephrotic Syndrome
of
Quartan Malaria

Nephrotic Syndrome of Quartan Malaria

John W. Kibukamusoke
M.D., F.R.C.P.(E), D.T.M. & H.

Professor of Clinical Medicine at Makerere University, Kampala; Chairman, National Research Council of Uganda; Formerly Chairman East African Medical Research Council; Formerly Senior Consultant Physician, Uganda Government

With a Chapter on Pathology by:

Professor M. S. R. Hutt, M.D., F.R.C.P., F.R.C.Path. Department of Morbid Anatomy, St. Thomas' Hospital Medical School, London, S.E.1. Formerly Professor of Pathology at Makerere University, Kampala

EDWARD ARNOLD

First published 1973
by Edward Arnold (Publishers) Ltd.,
25 Hill Street, London, W1X 8LL

ISBN: 0 7131 4197 2

Set in 11/12 pt. Monotype Plantin, printed by letterpress, and bound in Great Britain at The Pitman Press, Bath

Foreword

Although Professor Kibukamusoke's monograph on the *Nephrotic Syndrome of Quartan Malaria* opens with the statement that few diseases have been neglected as this one, he has nevertheless succeeded in marshalling an impressive series of references to relevant material. Beginning with Hippocrates in ancient Greece and particularly during the nineteenth and twentieth centuries, numerous observers in Europe, Asia, Africa and the Americas, have noted an association between renal pathology and malarial fever. As data accumulated and the focus became sharper, nephrosis and *Plasmodium malariae*—malaria—gradually emerged as the chief component factors in the syndrome.

Each aspect of the syndrome—historical, clinical, biochemical, parasitological and pathological—is described in turn in the monograph. (The chapter on Pathology is contributed by Professor M. S. R. Hutt.) All chapters lead, by separate pathways, to the main thesis, namely: that the aetiology of the nephrotic syndrome of quartan malaria is immunological; and that the deposition of complexes consisting of soluble plasmodial antigen and specific antiplasmodial antibody on the basement membrane of the glomerulus is the direct cause of the disease.

The author enlivens the text with numerous case histories from his own practice at Mulago Hospital, Kampala, Uganda. He also draws extensively on the experience of other workers, particularly in Africa. Since conflicting data are included in the text, the trend of the argument is not always directly linear, but exhibits the minor regressions and 'imperfections' which characterise biological data presented without bias.

The thesis that the nephrotic syndrome of quartan malaria is an immune condition is finally supported both by the direct demonstration of immune complexes in renal biopsies, and by the indirect therapeutic effect of immuno-suppressive drugs.

The monograph leads the reader from the intuitive vision of the earlier workers, through mounting conviction as facts accumulated, to final proof of the thesis. The history of the idea is given centre stage, and later work is shown to be firmly rooted in earlier studies. The continuity of the scientific effort in historical perspective emerges clearly; while it becomes equally clear that his own numerous contributions to the elucidation of this problem have given the author special authority to synthesise the scattered elements into an integrated whole.

It is a hallmark of ongoing research that each resolved problem raises new queries. Thus, for example, future studies will no doubt attempt to explain why *Plasmodium malariae* appears to be specifically associated with the nephrotic syndrome; while other plasmodia, also introducing soluble plasmodial antigen into the circulation, do not appear to be implicated in the syndrome to the same degree. Another field of study suggested by the monograph is the problem of renal pathology in the nonhuman malarious host. The few intriguing glimpses we are given into renal involvement in simian malaria suggest that suitable laboratory models studied in depth might well yield further insight into the human disease.

Much effort is perforce expended in preparing a critical historical review of a controversial subject. Future workers on the nephrotic syndrome in quartan malaria, using this review as a springboard, will owe a debt of gratitude to the author for bringing scattered and often puzzling units of information into an orderly and meaningful array.

February, 1971.

AVIVAH ZUCKERMAN
HEBREW UNIVERSITY
JERUSALEM, ISRAEL

Preface

Recent advances in the diagnosis and treatment of renal disease have stimulated a fresh wave of interest in human glomerulonephritis. But the extensive knowledge available from animal experiments could not be extrapolated directly with clinical material. With the recent studies in the nephrotic syndrome associated with quartan malaria a suitable human counterpart of the experimental disease became available. There is today a great deal of interest in this syndrome, so that a book devoted to the subject needs no further justification.

In 1963 Frank Dixon working in La Jolla, California, described the occurrence of immune deposits in the kidney of animals which had been given injections of a foreign protein. He showed that deposition occurred when soluble immune complexes formed in the circulation. This happened during conditions of a slight excess of antigen over antibody—a state of near equivalence which he termed 'an antigen-excess situation'. The process produced a proliferative glomerulonephritis. This observation has since been confirmed by a large number of workers and has been shown to occur in human disease: serum sickness, lupoid nephritis, poststreptococcal glomerulonephritis and, I believe, now the nephrotic syndrome of quartan malaria.

This book is the result of 10 years' work on the nephrotic syndrome of quartan malaria done mainly at Mulago Hospital, Kampala, Uganda. In addition the significant contributions from Nigeria have been reviewed and included.

I have attempted to make a comprehensive review of the available literature and to present pertinent information on the subject. In doing this I have deliberately gone into some detail on parasitology in order to provide in one place all available pointers to malaria as an aetiological factor. This approach seems to me infinitely justified for a relatively new subject such as this—a subject in which controversy inevitably exists. I can only hope that this approach will help to dispel some of the dissidence that currently exists on this subject particularly on the disease among adult patients.

The chapter on immunology is partly speculative and this has been done deliberately in order to stretch the readers' perception into the distant horizon and thus hope to stimulate further thought and work on this interesting problem. Identification of the antigen responsible for the vital immunological changes in this disease is currently the foremost problem. Experimental malaria has already begun to yield valuable information but the difficulty (in fact until recently, impossibility) of transmitting human plasmodia to experimental animals has been the biggest handicap. With the conquest of this problem it is to be hoped that the owl monkey, *Aotus trivirgatus*, will now provide us with a laboratory model of human *P. malariae* nephropathy. The 1970–80 decade should therefore hold much in stock for us in this field.

The demonstration of malaria parasitaemia still poses a formidable problem particularly among the adult cases, but as the parasite itself does not play a direct part in the production of glomerular damage identification of the antigen may sidestep this problem. However, as we still have to rely on the eye to identify the parasite through the microscope, I consider it desirable to include two plates in the text on the microscopic appearances of *Plasmodium malariae*. In thin slides the compact appearance of the parasite has been particularly useful and in thick slides, which are necessary for the demonstration of the light parasitaemias in this disease, the coarse malarial granules, produced by the parasite, have been a great help in its identification.

I wish to record my thanks to many people who have given selfless help and advice during the course of this work. It would be impossible for me to mention everybody here but those whom the limited space allows me mention are: first and foremost, Professor M. S. R. Hutt, formerly Head of the Department of Pathology at Makerere University and now of the Department of Morbid Anatomy at St. Thomas's Hospital Medical School, London, who has been a tower of strength to me. He has given me unflinching support throughout the entire course of this work. I am grateful to say that he has agreed to write Chapter 5 on pathology. Dr. A. G. Shaper, formerly Research Professor at Makerere and now of the Social Medicine Research Unit at the London School of Hygiene and Tropical Medicine has also given much valuable criticism and many suggestions. I am deeply thankful to him. Valuable suggestions are also acknowledged from Professor L. C. Bruce-Chwatt, Professor H. E. de Wardener, Professor A. W. Woodruff, Dr. A. Voller, Dr. A. J. Wing, Dr. N. E. Wilks and Professor George Nelson. I also acknowledge with grateful thanks the help I received from Dr. Peter A. Ward, then Chief of the Immunobiology Branch of the Armed Forces Institute of Pathology, Washington D.C., U.S.A., for immunoflorescence studies and also for Figs. 6.3–6.9, Dr. A. Voller for help with serum immunoglobulin studies, Professor J. Hardwicke for screening a number of sera for soluble immune complexes, Dr. A. C. Allison for Figs. 5.13 and 5.14, and the publishers of the following journals for permission to use Figures and Tables: *British Medical Journal, East African Medical Journal, Lancet* and *Military Medicine*. Research Grants were received from the World Health Organisation, Makerere University and the National Research Council for Uganda; for these I am very grateful.

Lastly but not least I am grateful to my wife, Sanyu, who put up with

the considerable inconvenience of burning the midnight oil and con-
finement to my desk during weekends and holiday periods. I wish also
to pay thankful tribute to the patience of our secretaries, notably Mrs. I.
Coelho, Mr. D. Sebadduka and Mrs. S. Andrades.

J. W. KIBUKAMUSOKE

Makerere University School of Medicine
Kampala, Uganda

January 1971

Contents

1   Historical Background

'. . . there was danger lest death should occur among young children and women and least of all among old people, and that the survivors should lapse into quartan fevers and from quartan fevers into dropsies. . . .'

Hippocrates.

Although the Nephrotic Syndrome of Quartan Malaria has been recognised since the times of Hippocrates and is an important cause of morbidity and mortality in tropical areas it has attracted little attention in the medical literature of the world.

A small number of dedicated workers, notably Rowland (1892), Giglioli (1930, 1962a, b) and Clarke (1912), have repeatedly, albeit unsuccessfully, called attention to the prevalence and significance of the disease. A quotation from Clarke (1912) will serve to illustrate this point:

'. . . I believe that the occurrence of oedema in the tropics of such a nature as to make one think of parenchymatous nephritis, is a reason for making a search for quartan malaria parasites imperative. . . . Every medical man knows that given the malaria parasite he may find albuminuria but he does not know that given the albuminuria without any fever he may find malarial parasites in over 50 per cent of the cases and of this 50 per cent almost 100 per cent is quartan.'

Giglioli (1930, 1932, 1962a, b) has been the champion of this disease through the last thirty years or so and it is to him that we owe much of our knowledge on the subject.

In every continent where malaria has existed someone has described a case of dropsy in whom he found quartan malaria parasites. It will be pertinent here to review the reports from the different continents pertaining to quartan malaria and the nephrotic syndrome.

Europe

Hippocrates' work in Greece has already been referred to. It described the occurrence of dropsy among women and children who survived many attacks of quartan fevers. The quotidian periodicity of the fever was a distinctive feature.

The earliest known report of proteinuria occurring during the intermittent course of malarial fever is said to have been given by Blackhall in 1818. Twenty-seven years later (1845) Chenouard recorded his conviction that many of the cases of nephritis and proteinuria, that he was seeing were due to 'intermittent fever'. Neret (1847) also described similar cases which he had encountered. A year later Martin Solon declared that proteinuria could be found in 25 per cent of all cases of 'intermittent fever'.

In his inaugural dissertation, Lenz (1865) claimed that 'intermittent fever' was a very frequent cause of diffuse nephritis.

In Germany, Rosenstein (1858) drew attention to the frequency of nephritis in malaria and in 1896 reported that 23 per cent of 162 cases of nephritis appeared to be malarial in origin.

Bartels (1877) in Ziemssen's Encyclopaedia lays great stress on malaria as a cause of chronic parenchymatous nephritis. He gives it as one of the most important causes in his experience. He writes: 'a not inconsiderable number of cases have been admitted into the hospital in this city during the last ten years, from the marshy districts bordering on the Elbe and the North Sea in Sleswick and Holstein, in which the grave renal disease had developed after long continued intermittent fever'. In the same paper he also reports the case of a 30 year old engineer who in 1873 contracted malaria for the first time while engaged in building a dyke at Jahdebusen. He suffered no febrile attacks but was admitted a few months later under Bartels' care with severe anasarca and gross proteinuria.

Hertz (1877) also confirmed the frequency with which proteinuria of considerable severity was found in cases of malaria. He wrote that protein was to be found in the urine not only on the fever days but also during the intermission and that some cases passed into a state of chronic diffuse nephritis.

In 1878, Soldatow reported a high incidence of renal disease in 350 necropsies of Russian soldiers dying of malaria in East Roumelia.

In France, Kelsch and Kiener (1889) gave a very good account of the clinical features of renal disease in 'malarial poisoning'.

In Italy, Rem-Picci (quoted by Giglioli, 1930) reported that in a study of malarial patients during the period 1891–1898 he found 80 cases with proteinuria ranging from 'plain albuminuria to established nephritis'. Thirty years later Patterni (1929) working in the same hospital studied 1,470 admissions for malaria. He found that the situation had changed and commented that 'with the progress of malaria control, with the greater facilities for early and efficient quinine treatment and hospitalisation of patients in suitable hygienic environment, kidney diseases of malaria origin, as other organic diseases depending from this infection, tend to become progressively mild and to acquire a transitory character'.

Marchiafava and Bignami (1902) reported a case of acute nephritis in whom quartan malaria parasites were found. After more extensive studies they concluded that renal damage in this form of malaria was due to some toxic substance which the blood stream brings to the kidney for elimination.

Few reports are available from England. Atkinson (1884) considers that this was due to the rarity of malarial illness in that country. Most of the reports related to the 'old Indians' (Britons who had lived in India for a long time) who had suffered from malarial fevers and died of chronic Bright's disease.

Asia

Watson (1905) reported a study of 83 cases of quartan malaria from Malaya. He observed that 50 per cent of them showed a moderate or severe degree of oedema and that all but five showed a heavy proteinuria. Some of the proteinuric patients showed chronic nephritis at necropsy. In some of the cases, however, both oedema and proteinuria disappeared on quinine therapy. In the same paper Watson reports that 18 per cent of the cases had no fever at any time and that a further 18 per cent showed a few spikes only separated by an average of 8·8 days.

Clarke (1912) in a vivid account from Malaya wrote that over 50 per cent of cases of nephritis show malaria parasites and that 'of this 50 per cent almost 100 per cent is quartan'. In a series of 62 cases of nephritis, only 5 of whom had fever, 29 showed P. malariae while three others showed other malaria parasites.

In 1927, Manson-Bahr and Maybury reported two cases of the nephrotic syndrome treated at the Hospital for Tropical Diseases, London. One was acquired in India and the other in Malaya. Both had P. malariae. Bosch (1930) reported cases of the nephrotic syndrome found in Java in association with malaria.

Surbek (1931a, b) described the features of an adult Javanese aged 24 who presented with the nephrotic syndrome in Sumatra. He found a very heavy infection with P. malariae. Parasitaemia cleared with quinine treatment but the nephrotic state persisted. The patient eventually died and at autopsy his kidneys showed normal looking glomeruli. Surbek reported a further eight cases he had encountered previously. Seven were children and one an adult.

Giglioli (1930) quotes James and Gunesekara's figures from the Port of Talaemannar in Ceylon. He also refers to Bahr's figures from another part of Ceylon. These figures were compiled in 1913. They show a high incidence of deaths from nephritis—about 25 per cent of deaths being due to this cause.

In the Solomon Islands and New Guinea James (1939) reported a study of 22 patients, 80 per cent of whom were under seven years of age, with severe oedema of the face, legs, and scrotum, a considerable degree of ascites and an enlarged 'malarial spleen' often extending below the umbilicus. The urine in these cases was loaded with protein. In fact they presented the clinical picture of the nephrotic syndrome. He found no urea retention or hypertension in any of them but malaria parasites were present in 8 of 15 of them, the majority showing the quartan variety. He stated that the patients were often chronic malarial subjects and that efficient treatment with quinine usually produced a rapid and dramatic recovery. He concluded that much of the nephritis, especially in children in those parts of the Pacific was of malarial origin.

Harrison and Dakin (1944) reported the case of a female native child from a south-west Pacific Island aged 5 years. This child was admitted in October 1943 to the Royal Australian Air Force hospital with severe nephrotic syndrome of one week's duration. A history of intermittent fever for several months was also obtained. There was no hypertension. The spleen was enlarged and the blood showed numerous *P. malariae* and *P. vivax* parasites. Proteinuria was profound. The child eventually became oedema-free on a good diet, bed rest and antimalarials. A moderate degree of proteinuria, however, persisted. These workers concluded that . . . 'in view of the well-known association between the two conditions (*P. malariae* and nephrotic syndrome) in other parts of the world and the "satisfactory" response to treatment it is considered that their combination in this patient was significant'.

Berger *et al.* (1967) reported three patients who developed acute glomerulonephritis on return from active service in Vietnam. All these patients developed oedema and showed heavy infections with *Plasmodium falciparum*. These workers considered that the acute nephritis was complicated by the nephrotic syndrome. This work is discussed further in Chapter 4 (p. 54).

North America

Woodward (1863) in his *Camp Diseases* stated that kidney disorder frequently complicated chronic malarial poisoning. Varying degrees of proteinuria were seen and some of the cases many of whom exhibited severe anasarca died of chronic renal disease.

Busey (1873, 1880) recorded a number of cases of renal disease in children, the origin of which he attributed to malaria. Da Costa (1881) similarly, reported that he had seen a large number of cases of Bright's disease following malaria.

A large number of other North American workers have also reported renal disease in association with malaria: Loving (1883); Berkley (1883); Pepper (1866) and Clemens (1880).

Atkinson (1884) published an extensive review of renal reactions in malaria. He also included details of his own observations on the subject. He quoted several cases where recurrent attacks of quotidian fevers led to the appearance of persistent proteinuria and dropsy. He also recorded observations on his own cases who progressed from the dropsical to the uraemic state in which they died despite quinine therapy. Oedema and proteinuria disappeared on quinine therapy in some of the cases which he had treated in the early stages of the disease.

Boyd (1940), observing the effect of quartan malaria as a therapeutic agent transmitted the parasite by mosquito bite or blood inoculation to 43 adults. He found that all developed proteinuria and that this was considerable in 14. Five individuals developed oedema of the lower extremities and one of these also had ascites.

Keitel *et al.* (1956) reported a case of the nephrotic syndrome due to congenital *P. malariae* infection in a 21 month old child who presented with the nephrotic syndrome after several months of irregular fevers. The mother was a narcotic addict who shared unsterilised syringes with other addicts. She was also shown to have an active *P. malariae* infection. The nephrotic syndrome completely remitted after a week's course of chloroquine.

South America

In a masterly treatise entitled *A contribution to the study of Bright's disease, as seen in Malarious countries* Rowland (1892) presented convincing evidence of a very high incidence of chronic nephritis and of a renal condition that is now called the nephrotic syndrome in British Guiana. He considered that chronic parenchymatous nephritis going on to secondary kidney contraction was very common and that it arose from 'intoxication paludéene aguë' and 'cachexie paludéene chronique' for the most part.

A few years later Daniels (1897) working in Georgetown (British Guiana) reported that the autopsy incidence of nephritis was 25 per cent. He found 228 cases with renal lesions among 926 consecutive malarial autopsies.

In nearby Surinam, Lambers (1932) examined 1,833 adult cases of malaria and found that 222 were infected with *Plasmodium malariae*. One hundred and nine of these (49·1 per cent) showed evidence of nephritis.

Swan (1909) dealing with the complications of malarial fevers reported that quartan malaria often complicated chronic parenchymatous nephritis.

In Panama, Bates (1913) demonstrated proteinuria in 42 per cent of cases of malaria.

In 1931 A. W. Grace and F. B. Grace were sent to Georgetown as a Special Commission to investigate what was then called 'the endemic nephritis of British Guiana'. Unfortunately most of their effort was devoted to other diseases and the disease they were commissioned to study is dismissed in a few sentences in the report. However they recognised two forms of kidney disease on histological grounds: parenchymatous nephritis and interstitial nephritis (this was the accepted terminology in those days). However they included a third: 'epidemic dropsy'. In all they studied 400 cases, 180 of whom were labelled epidemic dropsy, 172 parenchymatous nephritis and 48 interstitial nephritis. They went on to say that the developed disease (parenchymatous or interstitial nephritis) was identical in all respects, including chemical changes in the blood, with its counterpart in the temperature climates. Unfortunately they undertook no malaria parasitological studies.

The problem in British Guiana was clarified by Giglioli (1930). He found that the nephrotic syndrome was a very common form of renal disease and that a high proportion of deaths were due to chronic nephritis. He also found a very high incidence of symptomless proteinuria which was occasionally heavy in amount. Orthostatic proteinuria was also very common. He suggested that repeated attacks of malaria might eventually lead to persistent proteinuria. He also found that proteinuria was twice as common in quartan malaria as in other types of malaria and that there was a selective increase of *P. malariae* parasitaemia in cases of the nephrotic syndrome. He concluded that *P. malariae* was aetiologically connected with the endemic nephritis of British Guiana. In 1932 he reported the pathological findings in 5 fatal cases of the syndrome. The main changes in the kidney were those of chronic nephritis with secondary interstitial change in all but the very young.

In 1962*b* Giglioli presented further observations on the nephrotic syndrome and quartan malaria. These studies showed that there was a change in the pattern of renal disease during 10 years of malarial eradication. By the end of this period only 35,000 of the population of half a million remained exposed to endemic malaria, and this was only of moderate intensity. During the period of the 1920s the incidence of proteinuria in the population was 4·5 per cent and the annual incidence of chronic nephritis was 108 cases. By 1960 the incidence of proteinuria had fallen to 1·8 per cent and of chronic nephritis to a mere 7 cases. He also states that a diagnosis of nephrosis was never made during the latter period. He concluded that 'as the population in the area has trebled during the last 20 years, the virtual disappearance of chronic nephritis as compared with our figure for 1923–1929 is even more striking'.

Maegraith (1948) in his review of the literature on *Pathological processes in malaria and Blackwater Fever* stated that 'in acute malaria this nephrosis occurred mainly in *P. falciparum* infections, but in chronic or recurrent malaria it was commoner in *P. vivax* and *P. malariae* infections'. He considered that the differences between the pathological changes in the former infection and in the latter depended upon the more toxic activity of *P. falciparum* and the tendency for the other species to relapse and become latent. He however clearly distinguished between the changes of acute tubular necrosis occurring in association with acute *P. falciparum* infections and the glomerular changes of varying severity which may occasionally occur with *P. malariae* infections. He emphasised however that in *P. vivax* and *P. malariae* infections a sub-chronic nephritis developed and was succeeded in due course by a 'chronic parenchymatous' nephritis and ultimately by 'chronic interstitial' nephritis. He stated further that in the initial stages the changes were reversible and confined to albuminuria and passage of casts while later symptoms of hydraemic nephrosis supervened and finally gave place to those of uraemia.

Maegraith (1948) also quotes several other authors who described cases of 'hydraemic nephrosis' in whom malaria parasites, usually quartan, were found. The renal changes in 'many of the cases' reported showed a discrepancy between the severity of glomerular and tubular changes; the latter being much more severe than the former. He remarks however that there is general agreement amongst workers on the appearance of degenerative lesions but that few have recorded the diffuse cellular infiltrative and proliferative picture, or other severe glomerular changes such as were described by Giglioli (1932).

Maegraith (1948) also described a picture of acute nephritis as one of the four clinical types of renal reactions in malaria. He quotes Jansco and d'Engel's review (1931) of their experiences over 50 years in a clinic in Hungary. This report described fourteen out of 28 cases of acute nephritis in whom the nephritis appeared during the course of acute malaria. The offending parasite however was *P. falciparum*. Surbek (1931*a*, *b*), however, described one case out of 17 of this type which was associated with *P. malariae*. It is impossible without further information to be certain whether the finding of *P. malariae* in this case was not a mere coincidence. However, similar cases are quoted by James (1910) and Marchiafava and Bignami (1903). These were apparently cases of acute nephritis associated with gross oedema which occurred during the course of *P. malariae* infections. Maegraith also goes on to say that more rarely there may be 'a picture closely simulating the acute nephritis of streptococcal infections, with severe oliguria, nitrogen retention and uraemia'.

Middle East

In Palestine, Goldie (1930) studied a number of cases who presented with the nephrotic syndrome. He obtained a history of fever in all of them and published details of four of the most typical cases. He reviewed the literature up to that date and pointed out that descriptions of kidney changes in chronic recurrent malaria varied from 'big fat kidney' to 'small granular kidney'. He concluded that 'fatty changes and degeneration' of the tubules were the commonest findings, the pathological picture being that of a nephrosis of the hydraemic type.

Africa

In Ghana (then Gold Coast) McFie and Ingram (1917) reported nine cases of the nephrotic syndrome. These patients were all children under 10 years of age and *P. malariae* was demonstrated in blood slides from each one of them.

In Kenya, Carothers (1934) reported that 67 per cent of children with the nephrotic syndrome showed malaria parasites whereas only 8 per cent of the children without the syndrome showed parasites. He concluded that 'in so far as one can judge from the limited number of cases, it would appear that quartan malaria might be a factor in the causation of nephritis'.

McGregor *et al.* (1956) in their study of the effects of repeated malarial infections in protected and unprotected Gambian children observed one case in the unprotected group who developed a marked proteinuria during a heavy *P. malariae* infection. They considered that though the proteinuria could easily have been completely independent of the infection the possibility that it was a sequel to quartan malaria remained.

Gelfand (1957) reported that nephritis was common in the African. 'In some cases of nephritis, malaria appears to play a part in its production. *P. malariae* is the most common parasite found in malarial nephritis. Further, it is mainly seen in children.'

Trowell (1960) after reviewing the literature stated that 'this appears fairly conclusive evidence, but the time is ripe for the reassessment of this problem in Africa with the aid of renal biopsy. Meanwhile a strong case has been made that in certain areas of Africa quartan malaria can cause changes in the urine which suggest a special variety of glomerulonephritis. This term should be limited to those having a positive blood slide and a prompt clinical cure to antimalarial treatment or distinctive changes in the kidneys at post mortem'.

More recently in Nigeria, Gilles and Hendrickse (1963*a*) reported a comprehensive study of 113 nephrotic patients aged between 2 and 10 years. They found an overall incidence of 88 per cent for *P. malariae* among them. For comparison they examined 920 children seen at University College Hospital with various illnesses other than nephrosis, none of whom had taken antimalarial drugs. The incidence of *P. malariae* among them was 24 per cent. A similar rate of *P. malariae* infection (18 per cent) was found among 340 unselected children in villages close to Ibadan. *P. falciparum* rates, however, were similar in the three groups of children: 62 per cent among nephrotics, 70 per cent among non-nephrotic ill children and 56 per cent among village children. The usual preponderance of *Plasmodium falciparum* over *Plasmodium malariae* was therefore reversed in the nephrotic children—a finding similar to Giglioli's (1930). These workers further found that there was a forward shift of the peak incidence of childhood nephrosis from the age of two to the age of 5 to 7. This peak coincided with the peak incidence of malaria infection among children. They concluded that '. . . these epidemiological findings indicate a definite relationship between the nephrotic syndrome in Nigerian children and infection with *P. malariae*'.

White and Hutt (1964) were impressed with the frequency of the nephrotic state in their work at Mulago Hospital (East Africa). They described four cases of acute nephritis who presented with the nephrotic syndrome.

Garnham (1966) in his comprehensive treatise on malaria parasites and other Haemosporidia wrote that *P. malariae* had another and more serious effect—an attack on the kidneys leading to the severe 'quartan nephrosis'. He also went on to record his experiences of the condition in hospital practice at Kakamega in Kenya in 1935. He saw a whole ward occupied entirely by oedematous children, *all infected* with *P. malariae*.

The first comprehensive study of the nephrotic syndrome in Uganda was commenced in 1961 and was reported in 1966 and 1967. This showed the high incidence of the nephrotic syndrome both in children and adults and indicated that the disease was closely related to *P. malariae*. A comparison of the disease between Kampala, Uganda and Lagos, Nigeria, showed that it was similar in all respects (Kibukamusoke, 1966*a*).

In Lagos, Nigeria, the peak incidence of admissions for the nephrotic syndrome to the University of Lagos Teaching Hospital coincided with maximum rainfall for Lagos City and female anopheline densities for that city. This suggested that there was a common factor between them and the common factor seemed in all probability to be malaria. In agreement with our East African work (Kibukamusoke *et al.*, 1967; Kibukamusoke, 1968), I found a selective increase of *P. malariae* parasitaemia among patients with the nephrotic syndrome in Nigeria when I compared them with matched controls (Kibukamusoke, 1966*a*).

Malaria antibody studies also showed a significant increase in titre levels in the nephrotic group. In these papers much circumstantial evidence was given to show that the relationship between quartan malaria and the nephrotic syndrome was *causal* and concluded that an 'antigen excess' situation (Dixon, 1963) could account for the findings. Dixon postulated that circulating antigen—antibody complexes could damage the kidney.

Soothill (1967) has found evidence suggestive of the presence of these complexes. Studying Nigerian children with nephrosis he found that the majority showed proteinuria of moderate selectivity only using immuno-chemical differential protein clearances. By immunoelectrophoretic techniques he also found the altered form of complement component (βIC) in the serum obtained from children with poorly selective proteinuria. Similar findings have been made in other renal conditions where immune reactions are presumed to be taking place (Soothill, 1967). Soothill and Hendrickse (1967) further found that βIC normally present in the middle peak of Sephadex G-200 was detectable in the first peak which contains the large-size proteins. This suggested that large soluble complexes were probably present, reinforcing the idea that the disease is predominantly immunological in its mechanism.

The unusual degree of resistance to steroids (Kibukamusoke, Hutt and Wilks, 1967) and the supervention of the nephrotic state on conditions not usually associated with it (Kibukamusoke, 1966*b*; Kibukamusoke, Hutt and Wilks, 1967) led to the suggestion that this is probably a distinct form of the nephrotic syndrome and that it should be given a special designation—'the nephrotic syndrome of quartan malaria'.

Several workers have expressed dissatisfaction with the evidence for a causal relationship between malaria and the nephrotic syndrome. Atkinson (1884) mentioned several French and some German workers who did not agree that malaria could cause Bright's disease. Hirsch (1862), however, conceded that malaria was a cause in the very rare case. Atkinson (1884) believed that these dissident opinions were due to the fact that renal involvement varied greatly from one locality to another and that the actual incidence may depend on conditions of climate, soil, temperature, etc.

Atkinson's belief may be illustrated by Rosenstein's work (1858, 1896) who associated 23 per cent of cases of Bright's disease with malaria in Dantzic but encountered it with extreme infrequency in Gröningen, Northern Holland—then a fever province.

Raper (1953) studied a selection of 136 cases of renal disease derived from 2,800 autopsies. His conclusions were cautious because the study was retrospective with highly selected cases. It included only cases succumbing to renal disease. However, he stated that 'no evidence was obtained that renal disease in Uganda is attributable to malnutrition or malaria . . . '. Leather (1960) was also unconvinced, though he found malaria parasitaemia in 6 out of 12 children with 'glomerulonephritis'. He thought that 'this was a chance coincidence which would not be an unusual finding in a similar group of children in hospital in Kampala without nephritis in whom the blood was searched periodically, over a period of many weeks'. Unfortunately, he did not actually do this to a 'control' group. However, his three cases of acute nephritis (Leather, 1958) presented with the nephrotic syndrome. Leather (1960) was also very impressed with the severity of oedema in his cases of glomerulonephritis.

Renal reactions in artificially induced *P. malariae* infections

Boyd (1940) described a series of 43 psychiatric patients who were given quartan malaria infections for pyrexial therapy. Some were infected by mosquitoes and others by injection of infected blood. In 14 cases (33·5 per cent) proteinuria 'was at some time very heavy; so much that in 12 instances the onset of the complication made termination of the infection imperative'. Six patients developed oedema of the legs and in one of these the face and hands were also involved. In another ascites was present. In four the proteinuria was heavy though in two this was only a trace.

Boyd concluded that 'the most common incident in the clinical course of the infection was the development of an albuminuria which probably represents a nephrosis rather than a nephritis. This always cleared up with termination of the infection'. Unfortunately no histological studies are available as the technique for percutaneous renal biospy did not become available till 14 years later (Kark and Muehrcke, 1954).

The use of malaria in the treatment of the nephrotic syndrome

Paradoxically malaria has been used in the treatment of the nephrotic syndrome with some success. Shute (1952) recommended the use of only one species of plasmodia, *P. vivax*, because *P. falciparum* tends to produce very severe infections and *P. ovale* very ineffective ones. He excluded *P. malariae* because it tends to produce a very erratic infection after a long incubation period. The effects of artificially induced *P. malariae* infections in the nephrotic patient are thus unknown.

P. vivax has been used in most of the recorded cases, though *P. ovale* has been used occasionally. Gairdner (1952) treated 4 children with mosquito transmitted malaria and obtained an apparently full remission in two of them. In the remaining two no apparent benefit was observed. In this series the parasite species employed was given in one of the cases as *P. vivax*.

Byrne (1952) also treated a small boy of 2 successfully with mosquito transmitted *P. vivax*, while Porter (1954) achieved a similar result in a boy of 11.

Shaper (1955) reported 7 cases, three of whom derived prolonged benefit of freedom from oedema. Two cases, however, relentlessly progressed to death. In the remaining two the response was limited to partial control of oedema. *P. ovale* was used initially in one of the seven cases but as the febrile response was poor a *P. vivax* infection was subsequently induced.

Response to induced malaria therapy appears to be confined to diuresis though proteinuria has been reported to diminish in some cases. It is possible that the mechanism of response is based on endogenous stimulation of corticosteroid secretion during a febrile reaction, but there is as yet no direct evidence for this.

Conclusion

There would seem to be a convincing case for the association between quartan malaria and the nephrotic syndrome. We now have additional evidence to show that the relationship is of a 'cause and effect' type. In the chapters that follow details of the mechanism of damage and the resulting clinical picture will be given.

BIBLIOGRAPHY

Atkinson, I. E. (1884). Bright's disease of malarial origin. *Amer. J. med. Sci.*, **88**, 149.
Bartels, C. H. C. (1877). The structural diseases of the kidney and general symptoms of renal affections. *Ziemssen's Encyclop. Pract. Med.*, **15**, 1.
Bates, J. P. (1913). A review of a clinical study of malarial fever in Panama. *J. trop. Med. Hyg.*, **16**, 12, 177.
Berger, M., Birch, L. M. and Conte, N. F. (1967). The nephrotic syndrome secondary to acute glomerulonephritis during falciparum malaria. *Ann. int. Med.*, **62**, 6, 1163.
Berkley (1883). A case of transient albuminuria in malarial fever. *Maryland med. J.*, **10**, 227.
Bignami, A. (1903). L'infezione Malarica.
Blackhall, C. (1818). *Rec. mém. Med. Chir. Milit.*, **36**.
Bosch, W. G. (1930). Case of quartan nephrosis. *Gen. Ned.-Ind.*, **70**, 1101.
Boyd, M. F. (1940). Observations on naturally and artificially induced quartan malaria. *Amer. J. trop. Med.*, **20**, 749.
Busey (1873). Three cases of renal diseases in children, probably caused by malaria. *Amer. J. med. Sci.*, **65**, 123.
— (1880). Chronic Bright's diease in children caused by malaria. *Trans. Amer. med. Assoc.*, **31**, 715.

Byrne, E. A. J. (1952). Malarial therapy in lipoid nephrosis. *Lancet*, i, 844.

Carothers, J. C. (1934). An investigation of the etiology of subacute nephritis as seen among the children of North Kavirondo. *E. Afr. med. J.*, **10**, 335.

Chenouard (1845). *Rec. destrav. Soc. med. depart. d'Indre-et-Loire*, **101**, 1.

Clarke, J. T. (1912). Nephritis and quartan malaria. *J. trop. Med. Hyg.*, **15**, 133.

Clemens, J. M. (1880). Malaria with cases and remarks on renal complications. *Louisville med. News*, **10**, 145.

Da Costa (1880). Bright's disease as a result of exposure occurring in a malarial subject, as distinguished from the so-called malarial Bright's disease. *Med. Rec. (N.Y.)*, **17**, 54.

Daniels, C. W. (1897). Notes on postmortem examinations made in Public Hospital, Georgetown, from April 1895 to March 30th 1896. *Brit. Guiana med. Ann.*, **8**, 74.

Dixon, F. J. (1962–3). The role of antigen-antibody complexes in disease. *Harvey Lect.*, **58**, 21.

Gairdner, D. (1952). Nephrosis treated by malaria. *Lancet*, i, 842.

Garnham, P. C. C. (1966). In *Malarial Parasites and other Haemosporidia*. Blackwell, Oxford.

Gelfand, M. (1957). *The Sick African*, (3rd edition). p. 592. Juta, Cape Town.

Giglioli, G. (1930). *Malarial Nephritis*. Churchill, London.

— (1932). Clinical Notes, autopsy and histopathological findings from five fatal cases quartan malarial nephritis from British Guiana. *Trans. roy. Soc. trop. Med. Hyg.*, **26**, 177.

— (1962a). Malaria and renal disease, with special reference to British Guiana. I. Introduction. *Ann. trop. Med. Parasit.*, **56**, 101.

— (1962b). Malaria and renal disease, with special reference to British Guiana. II. The effect of malaria eradication on the incidence of renal disease in British Guiana. *Ann. trop. Med. Parasit.*, **56**, 225.

Gilles, H. M. and Hendrickse, R. G. (1963). Nephrosis in Nigerian children. Role of *Plasmodium malariae* and effect of antimalarial treatment. *Brit. med. J.*, ii, 27.

Goldie, H. (1930). Notes on association of malaria with nephritis. *Trans. roy. Soc. trop. Med. Hyg.*, **23**, 503.

Grace, A. W. and Grace, F. B. (1931). Researches in British Guiana 1926 to 1928. *Mem. London School Hyg. trop. Med.*, 3.

Harrison, K. S. and Dakin, W. P. H. (1944). Nephrotic type of nephritis in association with quartan malaria. *Med. J. Aust.*, **2**, 90.

Hertz (1877). Malarial diseases. *Ziemssen's Encyclop. Pract. Med.*, **2**, 641.

Hendrickse, R. G. and Gilles, H. M. (1963). Nephrotic syndrome and other renal diseases in children in Western Nigeria. *E. Afr. med. J.*, **40**, 186.

Hippocrates (Quoted by Giglioli, G. Malarial Nephritis, 1930).

Hirsch, A. (1862). *Handbuch der historisch—geographischen Pathologie*, Erlangen, **2**, 342.

James, C. S. (1939). Malarial nephritis (nephrosis) in Solomon Islands and mandated territory of New Guinea. *Med. J. Aust.*, **1**, 759.

James, S. P. and Gunesekara, S. T. (1913). Report on malaria at the Port of Talaemannar, Ceylon. *Govern. Rec. Off. Colombo*, **34**.

James, W. M. (1910). Quartan malaria and its parasite. *Proc. Canal Zone med. Assoc.*, **3**, 29.

Jansco, N. and d'Engel, R. (1931). Sur la néphrite dans le paludisome. *Riv. Malariol.*, **10**, 86.

Kark, R. M. and Muehrcke, R. C. (1954). Biopsy of kidney in prone position. *Lancet*, i, 1047.

Keitel, H. G., Goodman, H. C., Havel, R. J., Gordon, R. S. and Baxter, J. H. (1956). Nephrotic syndrome in congenital quartan malaria. *J. Amer. med. Assoc.*, **161**, 520.

Kelsch, A. and Kiener, P. L. (1889). *Traité des Maladies des Pays Chauds Region Pretropicale*. Bailliere, Paris.

Kibukamusoke, J. W. (1966a). The nephrotic syndrome in Lagos, Nigeria. *W. Afr. med. J.*, **15**, 6, 213.

— (1966b). *The nephrotic syndrome in Uganda with special reference to the role of Plasmodium malariae*. M.D. Thesis, University of East Africa, Kampala, Uganda.

— (1968). Nephrotic syndrome and chronic renal disease in the tropics. *Brit. med. J.*, **1**, 33.

Kibukamusoke, J. W., Hutt, M.S.R. and Wilks, N. E. (1967). The nephrotic syndrome in Uganda and its association with quartan malaria.*Quart. J. Med.*, **36**, 143, 393.

Lambers, J. A. (1932). Over Quartana-Nephritis en haar beteekenis in Suriname. *Geneesk. T. Ned. Ind.*, **72**, 334.

Leather, H. M. (1958). M.D. Thesis, University of Bristol, United Kingdom.

— (1960). Glomerulonephritis in Africans in Uganda. *Brit. med. J.*, **1**, 1930.

Lenz (1865). *Gryphiae*. De diffusa Nephritide Chronica, praecipue respecto decursu morbi post intermittentem febrim.

Loving (1883). Report of a case of intermittent fever complicated with acute albumunuria and general dropsy. *Med. J. Columbus* (i), 289.

Maegraith, B. G. (1948). *Pathological Processes in Malaria and Blackwater Fever*. Blackwell, Oxford.

Manson-Bahr, P. and Maybury, L. M. (1927). The association of quartan malaria with nephritis. *Trans. roy. Soc. trop. Med. Hyg.*, **21**, 131.

Marchiafava, E. and Bignami, A. (1902). *L'infezione Malarica*.

— (1903). *L'infezione Malarica*.

McFie, J. M. S. and Ingram, A. (1917). Observations on malaria in the Gold Coast Colony, West Africa. *Ann. trop. Med. Parasit.*, **11**, 1.

McGregor, I. A., Gilles, H. M., Walters, J. H., Davies, A. H. and Pearson, F. A. (1956). Effects of heavy and repeated malarial infections on Gambian infants and children. *Brit. med. J.*, **2**, 686.

Neret, D. (1847). Quelques observations de fièvres intermittentes avec albuminurie. *Arch. Con. Med.*, **15**, 509.

Patterni, L. (1929). Le nefropatic nella malaria. *Riv. malariol.*, **8**, 38.

Pepper, I. (1866). (i) Remittent fever; albuminous urine; pigment in blood; Death; pigment in all tissues of body. (ii) Remittent fever; death one and half hour after admission; pigment in brain, liver and spleen, etc., Albuminuria. *Amer. J. med. Sci.*, **51**, (i)–405 and (ii)–408.

Porter, R. (1954). Subacute oedematous nephritis treated with malaria. *Brit. med.J.*, **2**, 1398.

Raper, A. B. (1953). Nephritis and allied lesions in Central Africans. *E. Afr. med.J.*, **30**, 49.

Rosenstein, S. (1896). *Pathologie and Therapie der Nierenkrankheiten* (4 Anflage). Hirschwald, Berlin.

— (1858). Beitrag zur. aetiologie der parenchymatösen Nephritis. *Virchos arch.*, **14**, 110.

Rowland, E. D. (1892). Contributions to the study of Bright's disease as seen in malarious countries. *Brit. Guiana med. Ann.*, **4**, 41.

Shaper, A. G. (1955). Malarial therapy in the nephrotic syndrome. *Brit. med. J.*, **1**, 1132.

Shute, P. G. (1952). Malarial fever therapy. *Lancet*, ii, 333.

Soldatow (1878). *Petersburg Med. Wechenschr.*, No. 42.

Solon, M. (1848). Rôle de la rate dans les fièvres intermittentes. *Gaz. med.* (Sér 3), **3**, 618.

Soothill, J. F. (1967). *Clinical and Experimental Immunology*, Vol. 2. No. 1. Blackwell, Oxford and Edinburgh.

Soothill, J. F. and Hendrickse, R. G. (1967). Some immunological studies of the nephrotic syndrome of Nigerian children. *Lancet*, ii, 629.

Surbeck, K. E. (1931*a*). On renal reactions and nephritis in the course of malarial infections. *Trans. roy. Soc. trop. Med. Hyg.*, **25**, 201.

— (1931*b*). Complications of malaria. *Riv. Malariol.*, **10**, 194.

Trowell, H. C. (1960). *Non-infective Diseases in Africa*, p. 174. Edward Arnold, London.

Watson, M. (1905). Some clinical features of quartan malaria. *Indian med. Gaz.*, **40**, 49.

White, R. H. R. and Hutt, M. S. R. (1964). A clinico-pathological study of glomerulonephritis in East African children. *Arch. Dis. Childh.*, **39**, 313.

Woodward, J. J. (1863). Outlines of the chief camp diseases of the United States armies as observed during the present war. A practical contribution to *Milit. Med.*

2 Clinical Presentation and Natural History

The initial recognisable clinical expression of renal involvement in quartan malaria is by the nephrotic syndrome. This is true of all cases recorded in the literature from all parts of the world (reviewed in Chapter 1) and also of those cases who developed renal damage during the course of pyrexial therapy given for psychiatric disorders when *Plasmodium malariae* was the parasite used in treatment (Boyd, 1940).

Febrile proteinuria is well known in malaria and may occur during infection with each of the four species of human plasmodia. The frequency of febrile proteinuria in *P. malariae* infections, however, is reported to be higher than in any of the other three species, despite the fact that infection by *P. falciparum* produces the most severe clinical manifestations. This is illustrated by figures from Giglioli's *Malarial Nephritis* (1930).

Table 2.1

Parasite	Number of examinations	Number of cases with proteinuria	Percentage of cases with proteinuria (%)
P. Vivax	447	112	25
P. falciparum	67	14	20
P. Malariae	24	11	*46
Double infection	12	1	8

* The frequency of febrile proteinuria is significantly greater than with the remaining plasmodia (P < 0·05).

The prevalence of asymptomatic proteinuria in tropical populations is also very high. Giglioli (1930) reported the results of urine examinations in 9,510 apparently healthy young adults in British Guiana (Guyana). He found an average proteinuria rate of 4·5 per cent. However, rates up to 39 per cent were recorded in certain groups particularly after the malaria epidemic in Biritish Guiana (Guyana) of 1926 and 1927.

Heavy work precipitated proteinuria in a large number of subjects and it appeared to persist under the influence of continued manual labour (Giglioli, 1930). These observations probably relate to the state of malarial hyperendemicity and it is hard to imagine that this kind of proteinuria is not the precursor of the more severe lesions found in cases of the nephrotic syndrome and chronic nephritis so prevalent in the tropics (Kibukamusoke,1 968a). The lesions in febrile proteinuria may result from temporary deposition of soluble complexes on the renal basement membrane.

The syndrome produced generally conforms to the classical descriptions of the nephrotic syndrome (*Lancet*, 1959). Certain unusual or additional features, however, are often to be seen particularly among adult patients. These features are specifically attributable to concomitant histological changes in the kidneys.

These features will now be described in detail.

Oedema

Oedema has always been the presenting sign. It is progressive and usually makes the patient seek medical help. Its course is usually swift, from a rapid onset to a severe state of oedematous swelling. Its severity often suggests the diagnosis of the nephrotic syndrome at first sight. In about one-third of the patients the oedema is gross and may produce an appearance of neck retraction from severe submandibular oedema. Gross swelling of the eyelids may lead to complete closure of the eyes (Fig. 2.1). A large pad of sacral oedema is often present. In the most severe cases oedema fluid may be seen oozing through the tensely stretched skin of the lower limbs. With successful treatment the stretched skin retracts leaving striae on the thighs and abdomen and revealing the underlying cachexia which may be considerable. Oliguria is present in the majority of patients with severe oedema and ascites and twenty-four hour volumes of 250 to 500 ml. are not unusual. Pre-renal azotaemia is a common feature of the grossly oedematous patients. In some cases this factor aggravates established uraemia.

Ascites is almost invariably present (Fig. 2.1). It is severe in a large percentage of cases (Kibukamusoke 1968a) and is often very resistant to diuretic therapy. In the partially treated case the ascitic distension is often disproportionate to leg oedema and may lead to a false diagnosis of liver cirrhosis. Ascites is the last of fluid collections to disappear and may on occasion call for separate measures such as paracentesis abdominis. After this procedure it rapidly accumulates unless potent diuretics are concomitantly given.

Pleural effusions may be present but are rarely large enough to produce symptoms or necessitate special measures. Pericardial effusions are unusual though they have rarely been known to produce cardiac embarrassment. Pleural and pericardial effusions are usually proportional to the severity of oedema elsewhere in the body.

Proteinuria

Proteinuria is usually heavy. In a series of eighty cases (Kibukamusoke, Hutt and Wilks, 1967) 86 per cent showed a protein excretion ranging

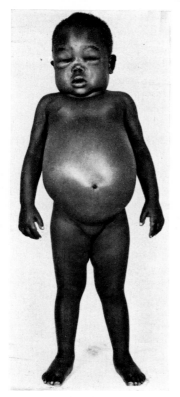
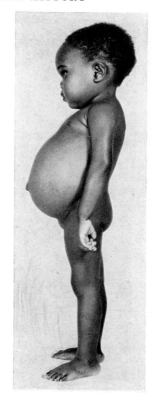

Fig. 2.1   Fig. 2.2

from 5 to 20 g in twenty-four hours. The average for the entire group was 7 g in the day. Squire (1960) showed that a loss of this magnitude (7 g) was capable of producing the nephrotic syndrome in small-sized patients. The presence of oedema and other features of the nephrotic syndrome could therefore be adequately accounted for by the severity of proteinuria in these cases.

In 11 cases (13·7 per cent) in this series protein was, however, excreted in quantities less than 7 g per day, but the variability of protein excretion and the period of time that expired before presentation make it difficult to assess the significance of this observation.

In an investigation of protein loss in the bowel in this condition two cases were studied using [131]I—labelled human albumen. We found that a loss was undoubtedly taking place in the bowel but the impression gained was that it was not a very great one. It is possible, of course, that the loss is sometimes heavy enough to augment the effect of relatively moderate urinary losses and thus precipitate the nephrotic state. No firm opinion can be given on this at the moment and further work needs to be done.

Protein undernutrition is well known in the tropics and marginal levels of albumen in the serum have been reported in otherwise normal individuals.

(Holmes *et al.*, 1951 and 1955; Leonard *et al.*, 1965). It is therefore possible that urinary protein loss of a moderate severity only may produce a severe enough hypoalbumineaemia to precipitate a nephrotic state. More work is also required on this point. The weight of evidence so far available, however, supports the possibility that loss through the urine is the principal factor in the lowering of serum albumen and the precipitation of the nephrotic syndrome in these patients.

The urinary deposit

Casts are usually present in freshly passed urine. They, however, break up very quickly if the urine is left to stand for a long time before examination. The frequency of highly alkaline urines in tropical populations (Kibuka-musoke, 1968*b*) enhances this disintegration. However, all forms of casts are met with, particularly the granular type (Kibukamusoke, Hutt and Wilks, 1967).

White cells are usually found in small numbers. In those cases where large numbers of white cells are found it is wise to look for further evidence of active pyelonephritis although absence of this and indeed of white cells does not completely exclude it.

Red cells are also found in small numbers and these may give a positive reaction for occult blood on the LABSTIX (Ames Company) test. Severe glomerular lesions of the proliferative type may be associated with heavier erythrocyte deposits and even red cell casts (Kibukamusoke, Hutt and Wilks, 1967).

Fever

It is unusual to see the nephrotic syndrome either during or after an acute attack of fever due to *P. malariae,* nor is fever a feature of the active phase of the nephrotic syndrome. This fact makes the timing of blood examination for parasites very difficult and very often parasites are recovered unexpectedly even when the infection is heavy. The following case will illustrate this point:

N., a Ganda female child aged 6 years, was admitted to hospital with severe oedematous swelling of the whole body. This had been progressive over the previous week. There was no history of fever during the past few months, nor was there any during her entire stay in the hospital (six weeks). Twenty thick blood slides were taken over a period of 72 hours (at 4-hourly intervals) for malaria parasites. Numerous *P. malariae* parasites were found in each one. There was gross proteinuria and serum biochemistry was consistent with a diagnosis of the nephrotic syndrome. Parasitaemia would have been missed in this case had one been looking for parasites in febrile cases only.

Classical quartan fevers have, however, been occasionally seen during the acute phase of the nephrotic syndrome, but this is by no means common.

Another situation which is also fairly commonly seen is the intermittent appearance of *P. malariae* in the blood. In such cases even the most diligent search of blood for malaria parasites either by the serial or sessional methods (Kibukamusoke, 1967*b*) will fail to demonstrate them. The following case will serve to illustrate this point:

R.N. a Ganda female child of 7 years of age was admitted to hospital with steroid-resistant nephrotic syndrome. She had been receiving treatment at a Mission Hospital nearby for a period of 6 weeks. No antimalarials had been given and no fever had been noticed either on admission, during the stay nor in the months preceding admission to the Mission Hospital. She stayed for 3 months with us during which period there was no exposure to malaria infection. Three previous 10-day searches for malaria parasites with a week's interval in between the searches had failed to reveal parasites. One day during the third month of her stay in our hospital she suddenly appeared off-colour, lost her appetite and vomited once. Her temperature rose slightly to 99° F (37·2° C). There was no evidence of a pyogenic infection anywhere and her white blood count was normal. A thick slide taken then, however, showed *P. malariae* parasites. This child therefore had *Plasmodium malariae* in her body all the time though they could not be demonstrated. It is likely that parasites were truly absent from the blood and only appeared during or to cause this episode of ill-health. The parasite was most probably sitting dormant in the liver in its exoerythrocytic phase.

This episodic appearance of parasitaemia has been seen on a number of other occasions and it may well explain the failures in the recovery of parasites which have been reported by several workers. A small rise of the temperature to 99° F (37·2° C) is easily missed, particularly if it is accompanied by very mild constitutional symptoms or perhaps none at all.

Any or all of the other clinical features constituting the nephrotic syndrome (*Lancet*, 1959; Arneil, 1961) may be present. When the glomerular changes are minimal the clinical presentation is that of the pure nephrotic syndrome (*Lancet*, 1959; Arneil 1961), but with more severe degrees of glomerular damage additional clinical features may be present. These are: hypertension, retinopathy, congestive cardiac failure and haematuria. These features will now be described.

(a) Hypertension

In a series of 80 consecutive cases of the nephrotic syndrome from all causes in Mulago Hospital (Kibukamusoke, 1966*a*) there were 34 cases with an associated hypertension. This was diagnosed when the diastolic pressure exceeded 100 mmHg under basal (resting) conditions. Among children under the age of 10 years levels above 70 mmHg and 80 mmHg for older children (10–14 years) taken under similar conditions were similarly interpreted.

Table 2.2 shows the histological diagnoses of the cases who showed hypertension.

Table 2.2

Histological diagnoses in hypertensive cases

Histological diagnosis	Number of cases
Focal glomerulonephritis	2
Generalised proliferative including membrano- proliferative glomerulonephritis	24
Membranous glomerulonephritis	1
Pyelonephritis	1
Renal vein thrombosis	1
Renal amyloidosis	1
Chronic nephritis	3
Henoch–Schöenlein syndrome	1
Total	34

In a review of 51 cases of the nephrotic syndrome associated with quartan malaria, hypertension was found in 18 cases (35 per cent) (Kibukamusoke, 1967a). Table 2.3 gives the details of this study.

Table 2.3

Occurrence of hypertension in 51 consecutive cases

Glomerular lesion	Total number	Number of children	Number with hypertension
Generalised proliferative glomerulonephritis	28	8	15 (53%)
Focal glomerulonephritis	9	6	2
Total	37	14	17 (33%)

51

It will be seen that a number of adults and some children have hypertension and that this is particularly associated with severe glomerular lesions of a proliferative type. Hypertension appears to contribute to the deterioration in glomerular structure and function that occurs in many of these cases.

Occasionally cases appear to present primarily with hypertension, particularly in the young adult. It is possible these derive from the group with persisting proteinuria (p. 29). An investigation into the causes of hypertension in fifteen young pregnant women in Kampala (MacSearraigh et al., 1969) showed that nine had the changes of proliferative glomerulo-nephritis on renal biopsy and some of these probably had a quartan malarial aetiology.

Examination of a clean specimen of urine is usually sufficient to confirm the renal origin of hypertension in these cases though renal function studies may be necessary in some. We have found renal biopsy to be a very useful investigation in this connection, though it is not absolutely necessary for the management of an individual case. Severe glomerular changes are usually associated with definite abnormalities in the urine and abnormal renal function tests. A fairly good idea can thus often be obtained by simple examination of the urine together with simple tests of renal function.

Less severe glomerular changes may not, however, be associated with abnormal function tests and this is the type of situation for which renal biopsy is particularly useful. Examination of the urine, however, is very often of great value as urinary abnormalities are almost invariable, particularly proteinuria. Proteinuria should never, even in traces be disregarded. A 24-hour specimen is useful in doubtful cases where trace amounts of protein are found in casual specimens.

Very mild cases may have truly intermittent proteinuria, and this may be precipitated only by exercise or manual labour. Proteinuria may therefore be missed under resting conditions and hypertension may under the circumstances appear to be primary.

The reliability of hypertension as an index of renal damage has been shown to be very low (Kibukamusoke, 1967a), and urea retention may be more reliable.

The most reliable figure to use as indicative of hypertension in the adult is 100 mmHg of diastolic pressure. Figures below this occur in other renal lesions which are not classically associated with hypertension.

(b) Retinal changes

This is found in about 12 per cent of cases and it is related to hypertension (Kibukamusoke et al., 1967). The severity of retinal lesions provide a good guidance to the rapidity of deterioration particularly if much chronic change is present in the glomeruli. Adequate control of hypertension is accompanied by reasonable regression of the retinal changes. Papilloedema is sometimes seen in these cases and once present the prognosis is very much worse (Wing, 1969).

(c) Congestive cardiac failure

This is usually secondary to hypertension. When present it is often the reason which brings the patient to the hospital.

In a study of 80 cases of the syndrome (Kibukamusoke, Hutt and Wilks, 1967) hypertension was present in 34 of the cases (42·5 per cent). In this series 58 per cent of all cases with a diastolic pressure of 95 mmHg or above showed severe proliferative glomerulonephritis.

Dyspnoea is a prominent feature in those cases where heart failure has supervened. The increase of oedema may not be obvious enough to compel the patient to seek medical aid but dyspnoea will often do.

In the 34 cases who had hypertension in a series studied by Kibukamusoke (1966a) the presenting complaint was dyspnoea in 14 cases. This symptom was due to congestive cardiac failure in every case.

Endomyocardial fibrosis is seen in some patients who have suffered or are actively suffering from this form of the nephrotic syndrome, but no accurate figures are available yet. It is possible that the association is purely coincidental, but it is equally possible that this is due to sharing a common pathogenesis. This point needs to be studied further particularly as it might throw some light on the aetiology of endomyocardial fibrosis, at present obscure.

(d) Haematuria

Haematuria is an almost invariable feature of the nephrotic syndrome of quartan malaria. It is related to the histological changes found in the glomeruli of affected individuals. This change is basically one of endothelial/mesangial cell proliferation. Bleeding is usually mild in degree and is generally confined to the presence of red cells in the urinary deposit. In my own series (Kibukamusoke, 1966a) all cases showed some red cells in the urine except three. The reason for the absence of red cells in these three cases was not clear, nor were glomerular changes different from those shown by the rest of the cases.

Haematuria may be severe enough to be noticed by the patient. Again in my personal series (Kibukamusoke, 1966a) six cases gave a history of haematuria. This was gross in two of the patients and repeated up to six times in two others. Recurrent haematuria of this type is reminiscent of focal glomerulonephritis (Ross, 1960). The histology in many patients is truly focal. It is not, however, intended to suggest here that these two syndromes are similar but only to point out some relevant similarities. The clinical picture is also similar in some patients in that a proportion of them remain apparently static (without deterioration or going into a full remission) for many years. It is possible that these are some of those whom Giglioli (1930) found to have proteinuria during a physical fitness examination for prospective employees on sugar estates in British Guiana.

Haematuria is truly glomerular in origin. Kibukamusoke et al. (1967)

found some red cell casts in the urine of some patients. Renal biopsies may also show red cells in the tubules in some of these cases.

The sudden occurrence of haematuria and oedema in some patients may lead to confusion with acute nephritis. The concurrent appearance of the nephrotic syndrome with this state has led to the term 'acute nephritis with the nephrotic syndrome'. Whilst this combination is not unknown in post-streptococcal glomerulonephritis (Wilson and Heymann, 1959), it is particularly suggestive of the nephrotic syndrome of quartan malaria in tropical practice.

Urinary volume

It is not unusual to come across 24-hour urinary volumes below a litre in hospital practice in the tropics. Total daily volumes in the nephrotic syndrome, however, are exceptionally small. The usual figures are 300–500 ml a day. This may in some cases be related to low renal perfusion rates consequent upon a contracted circulatory volume in severe oedematous states. Effective diuretic therapy often increases the daily volumes to 3 or 4 litres. Renal function may also improve with adequate diuresis.

Pregnancy

Pregnancy often worsens the nephrotic state and renal function. Oedema was aggravated in all of our pregnant cases (Kibukamusoke, Hutt and Wilks, 1967). While there was a remission of oedema after each of the first two pregnancies it tended to persist and force the patient to hospital after the third pregnancy.

Recurrence of oedema usually occurs during the third trimester. It may thus be very difficult to differentiate from toxaemia of pregnancy. Biochemical changes, however, will often be distinctive for the nephrotic state.

Other features

Age

(a) Children

In Europe and North America the peak incidence of the nephrotic syndrome in children has been observed to occur between the ages of 6 months and 2 years (Barnett, Forman and Lauson, 1952; Lawson, Moncrieff and Payne, 1960; Arneil, 1961). White et al. (1970) in an analysis of European cases in London revealed the existence of a peak in the immediate pre-school period (Fig. 2.3). Arneil (1961) had previously demonstrated a peak at an earlier age which was related to the use of mercury-containing teething powders. This factor is, of course, much less common today as teething powders no longer contain mercury.

In Africa a single large peak occurs at the age of 5–7 years (Fig. 2.4).

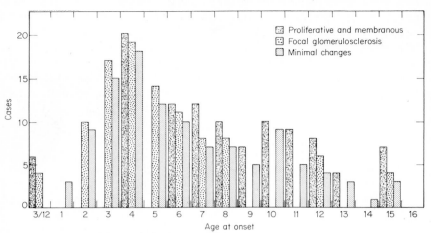

Fig. 2.3. Nephrotic syndrome: age incidence and renal morphology
(After White R. H. R., Glasgow E. F. and Mills J. R. 1970.
Lancet, **i**, 1353)

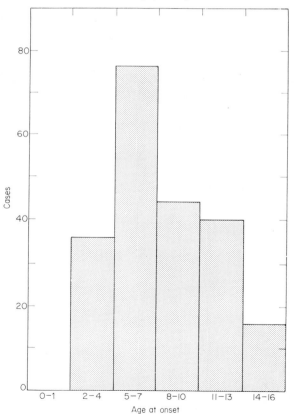

Fig. 2.4. Incidence of nephrotic syndrome in
childhood in Uganda (212 cases)

It will be seen that this peak is shifted forward to coincide with that of peak malaria infection in children (Fig. 4.6). All pointers suggest that this shift is caused by malaria. Later it will be shown that malaria is also responsible for the large numbers (height of peak) encountered in the tropics. Gilles and Hendrickse (1963) reported similar findings. The situation is probably true of the rest of the tropical countries.

(b) Adults

One of the most striking features of adult tropical medical practice is the frequency of chronic nephritis in young adults. This has been considered to be the result of progressive renal disease of malarial origin (Kibukamusoke, 1968a; Edington, 1967).

In a study of 80 cases (31 children and 49 adults) Kibukamusoke (1966a) found that 33 of these cases belonged to the age group 15–35 years (Fig. 2.5). This reveals a considerable waste of man power at a very active period of a person's life.

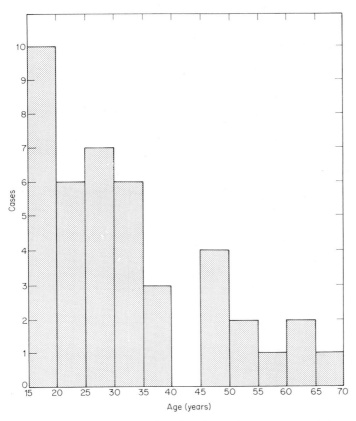

Fig. 2.5. The incidence of nephrotic syndrome among adults

Sex

In children under the age of 14 years the sex incidence was equal (Kibukamusoke, 1966a). The sex ratio was strongly weighted in favour of males in the adults. Figures suggest that this is merely a reflection of hospital sex admission ratios and not a true difference of sex incidence. Table 2.4 illustrates this point.

Table 2.4

Sex incidence among adult nephrotics

Age group	Females	Males
15–20	7	4
21–25	3	4
26–30	2	7
31–35	2	5
36–40	–	–
41–45	–	–
46–50	2	2
51–55	–	2
56–60	1	–
61–65	1	1
66 and over	–	1
Total	18	31
Grand total	49	

Tribal distribution

A detailed analysis of my own study (Kibukamusoke, 1966a) reveals that 78 subjects were of African stock. The main tribal distribution is given in Table 2.5.

Table 2.5

Tribal distribution

	Male			Female		
	Ganda	Rwandan	Others	Ganda	Rwandan	Others
Children (<15 yr.)	7	1	8	3	2	7
Adults	10	11	11	7	1	10
Totals	17	12	19	10	3	17

If these numbers are expressed as percentages of admissions during the period in which the study was done the following figures are derived for purposes of comparison (Table 2.6).

Table 2.6

Actual cases expressed as a percentage of admissions

| | Ganda | | Rwandan | |
	Male	Female	Male	Female
Children (1–14 yr.)	0·77	0·40	0·56	1·71
Adults (>15 yr.)	0·47	0·64	1·66	0·61

These figures show that the observed differences in percentage is more than twice the standard error of the difference between the Rwandan adult males (1·66 per cent) and Ganda adult males (0·47 per cent). This analysis suggests that adult male Rwandan subjects are significantly more prone to this form of the nephrotic syndrome than the Ganda male adults.

Shaper (1968) in a study of the immunology of people native to the central hyperendemic (malarial) region of Uganda (Baganda) and Rwandan migrants to this area, from an area of low malarial endemicity found that the latter had significantly higher malaria antibody titres than the former (see Table 2.7). These higher titres were associated with considerable

Table 2.7

Autoantibodies among Ganda and Rwandans

Malaria antibody titre	Ganda %	Rwandans %	IgM	Heart anti- bodies %	Thyroid anti- bodies %	Parietal cell anti- bodies %	Rheuma- toid factor %
1:400 or less	85	25	+	11	7	3	5
1:800 or more	5	75	+++	54	31	21	40

(From Shaper A. G. (1968). E. Afr. med. J. 45, 219.)

increases in the immunoglobulin IgM. The increases were also associated with a high incidence of autoantibodies to heart, thyroid, gastric parietal cells and the rheumatoid factor, though there was no overt evidence of disease affecting these organs.

Abnormal responses are therefore to be expected to occur pre-eminently among Rwandans, and the tribal analysis presented strengthens further the possibility of an immunological basis to the nephrotic syndrome of quartan malaria. It is important to note, however, that no tribal group is exempt— only an excessive prevalence among the immigrant Rwandans.

Growth retardation

Definite growth retardation has been observed in children with severe and prolonged disease. Several striking examples of this have been seen. One patient was a girl of 14 who had been affected since the age of 5. Her stature conformed to that of a girl of 9. Her hair was scanty and wiry and her skin was thin and cracked easily. Secondary sex characteristics were absent.

Effective treatment produces a remarkable spurt of growth in these cases and many of the abnormalities in skin and hair revert to normal. The patient described above soon developed secondary sex characteristics on institution of effective therapy. In our experience at the Renal Clinic, Mulago Hospital, Uganda, continuous malaria prophylaxis has had particularly striking effect on growth rates in these patients.

Relapses of the nephrotic state

These have been observed to follow a large variety of insults: re-infection with *Plasmodium malariae*, attacks of *P. falciparum* in two or three cases, viral or coryzal illnesses, pregnancy and mumps. A significant number have also relapsed without any apparent reason.

The combined picture of nephritis and nephrosis

Additional features of azotaemia, hypertension, and haematuria may be present. In the child these are uncommon but when seen they accompany an acute onset and thus warrant a description of 'acute nephritis with nephrotic syndrome'.

In the adult the combined picture is the rule rather than the exception. It is regularly associated with severe or progressive proliferative glomerulonephritis. Its presence in the patient therefore often permits a correct forecast of the pattern of histology in the glomeruli, which in turn determines the fatal outcome of the severe case (Wing, Hutt and Kibukamusoke, 1972 in press).

Pyelonephritis with the nephrotic syndrome

Pyelonephritis is not an accepted cause of the nephrotic syndrome. In Europe and North America pyelonephritis is known to complicate glomerulonephritis and this may have been associated with the nephrotic syndrome. In diabetes mellitus renal involvement may produce the nephrotic syndrome and pyelonephritis may be superimposed because susceptibility to infection is increased in diabetes mellitus.

In Uganda the association of oedema with pyelonephritis (particularly due to urethral stricture) is not uncommon. In the majority of cases the oedema is due to hypertensive cardiac failure but there remains a significant number of cases in whom the oedema is due to the nephrotic syndrome.

Kibukamusoke (1966b) reported two cases he had encountered in his studies of the nephrotic syndrome. In both cases long-standing pyelonephritis was undoubted. The patients had obstructive uropathy from chronic urethral stricture. Significant bacillary counts were obtained in both cases by culture of the urine, and pyelonephritis was confirmed by renal histology. Both cases showed patchy involvement of both kidneys by changes ascribable to pyelonephritis. Proteinuria was gross in both cases: 10 g/day in one case and 10–15 g in the other. Examination of the blood revealed all the biochemical changes of the nephrotic syndrome. There was thus no doubt that pyelonephritis and the nephrotic syndrome occurred concurrently in these two patients. The urethral strictures had been present for many years and one of the cases had established urinary fistulae. It was thus obvious that the pyelonephritis has preceded the nephrotic syndrome. One of the cases showed *P. malariae* in his blood and his serum malaria antibodies were very high (1 : 3,200).

Careful examination of histology sections from the 'non-involved' areas of the kidneys revealed normal-looking glomeruli but showing hyaline droplet change—indicating gross leakage of protein, in one case. In the other, the glomeruli were swollen and showed changes of acute endothelial cell proliferation. The tubules showed hyaline droplet change.

Gross protein leakage was therefore taking place through glomeruli uninvolved by pyelonephritis. This suggested that a separate factor was responsible for the leakage of protein and probably the nephrotic syndrome. Concurrent infection with *P. malariae* presents one possibility and a very likely one too though it is hard to prove. It is possible of course that as both the nephrotic syndrome, urethal strictures and malaria are all common in this environment the combination is fortuitous. This problem requires more extensive and carefully planned studies but until these are done the possibility of pyelonephritis causing the nephrotic syndrome, with *P. malariae* as a potentiator, remains.

Natural history

The natural history of the disease falls into the following groups:

1. A stable remission which develops spontaneously or with the use of immuno-suppressive drugs.
2. A remission of temporary duration only. The subsequent course may vary greatly from case to case.
3. Persistent proteinuria after an initial stage of classical nephrotic syndrome. Proteinuria may persist for many years without apparent clinical or histological deterioration.

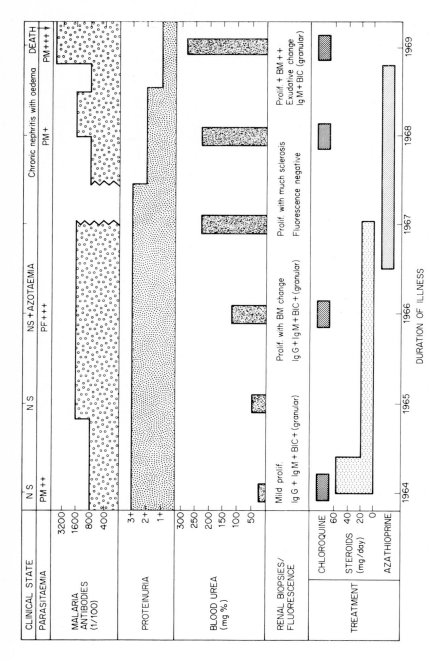

Fig. 2.6. N.M. female, aged 10 at onset, Rwandan—clinical data of a progressive case

NS Nephrotic syndrome   PM/PF *Plasmodium malariae/falciparum*
BM Basement membrane

4. A slowly progressive course to chronic hypertensive/azotaemic nephritis in early adulthood (Fig. 2.6).
5. A rapid course to early death in uraemia.

The classical picture in the adult is one of a mixture of the nephrotic syndrome and chronic renal failure. Progression from the nephrotic to the nephritic state is commonly observed and this is associated with loss of oedema. Thus a large number of adult patients give a past history of oedematous swelling or nephrotic state, although they present with established chronic nephritis. The author has observed a number of patients passing from the state of nephrosis to one of chronic nephritis and a proportion of these have died in uraemia.

In children a pure nephrotic state is usual but progression may occur in a small number to a non-oedematous state of chronic nephritis.

The following case history will serve to illustrate the above:

M.N. a female Rwandan aged 10 was admitted in August 1964 with severe nephrotic syndrome of 4 weeks' duration. She had a fever of 99°F (37·2° C) and a positive blood slide for *P. malariae*. The spleen was enlarged to 3 finger-breadths below the costal margin. Her blood urea was 25 mg per cent and the serum cholesterol was raised. A.S.O.T. was 1:100. Renal biopsy showed changes of proliferative glomerulonephritis and heavy granular or beaded deposits of IgM and βIC together with lighter deposits of IgG. The malaria antibody titre was 1:800 (using the indirect fluorescent technique of Voller and Bray, 1962). She was treated with diuretics and antimalarials and was discharged on malaria prophylactics to the follow-up clinic free of oedema. Proteinuria, however, continued.

Two months later her blood urea was 34 mg per cent though her serum cholesterol was normal. She unfortunately attended the follow-up clinic very irregularly except during the first 6 months when she was definitely better and put on several inches in height. After this initial period of improvement she turned up only when she had a fresh attack of malaria (usually *P. falciparum*) or on recurrence of oedema. Proteinuria continued to be heavy and 2 years later her blood urea was found to be 160 mg per cent. She required hospitalisation on 2 occasions during this period.

After a while she no longer required diuretics for the control of her oedema and this soon disappeared completely. The blood urea at this time was 236 mg per cent and the creatinine clearance 4 ml/min. She also had a hypertension of 130/110. The blood urea remained at this level till a few months before her last admission when it started to mount up again after a fresh infection with *P. malariae*. The blood pressure was 180/140. She died with a blood urea of 340 mg per cent, a serum creatinine level of 16 mg per cent and a terminal subdural haematoma. Her A.S.O.T. never exceeded 1:100 during this period.

Her kidneys were small and contracted at necropsy and histology showed proliferative glomerulonephritis with much glomerular scarring and atrophy (See Fig. 2.6 for clinical details).

Chronic renal failure is very common in the tropics and this is particularly striking among young adults. MacSearraigh *et al.* (1969) showed that the basis for many of the post-partum hypertensive cases they studied was proliferative glomerulonephritis and the lesions they found were similar to those we have associated with quartan malarial nephropathy. The widespread occurrence of quartan malarial nephrotic syndrome and the capability of the underlying renal lesion for progression seems to be the reason for this. A decline in the incidence of both the nephrotic syndrome and chronic renal disease has been observed to follow the eradication of malaria (Giglioli, 1962a, b).

Big spleen disease in patients with the nephrotic syndrome of quartan malaria

Big spleen disease is a syndrome found in many malarious countries. The evidence at present available points to quartan malaria as a probable cause (Marsden *et al.*, 1965). It is thought that the disease is caused by abnormal immunological reactions occurring in the semi-immune state of malaria, but the nature of these reactions has not been elucidated. The diagnostic histological changes consist of hepatic sinusoidal lymphocytosis and Kupfer cell hyperplasia.

As the nephrotic syndrome of quartan malaria has been shown to be due to abnormal immunological reactions occurring in *P. malariae* infections one would expect that some of the cases might show evidence of big spleen disease. In an analysis of 79 adult cases only 5 had big spleen disease. This frequency would be expected in a non-selected population in a hyperendemic malarious area. The disease does not therefore appear to be commoner among cases of quartan malaria nephrosis. This, however, is only an impression and properly controlled studies will be required to confirm or refute this conclusion.

BIBLIOGRAPHY

Arneil, G. C. (1961). One hundred and sixty four children with nephrosis. *Lancet*, ii, 1103.
Barnett, H. L., Forman, C. W. and Lauson, H. D. (1952). The nephrotic syndrome in children. *Adv. Paediat.*, **5**, 53.
Boyd, M. F. (1940). Observations on naturally and artificially induced quartan malaria. *Amer. J. trop. Med.*, **20**, 749.
Edington, G. M. (1967). Pathology of malaria in West Africa. *Brit. med. J.*, **1**, 715.
Giglioli, G. (1930). *Malarial Nephritis*. Churchill, London.
— (1962a). Malarial and renal disease, with special reference to British Guiana. I. Introduction. *Ann. trop. Med. Parasit.*, **56**, 101.

Giglioli, G. (1962b). Malaria and renal disease, with special reference to British Guiana. II. The effect of malaria eradication on incidence of renal disease in British Guiana. *Ann. trop. Med. Parasit.*, **56**, 225.

Gilles, H. M. and Hendrickse, R. G. (1963). Nephrosis in Nigerian children, role of *Plasmodium malariae*, and effect of antimalarial treatment. *Brit. med. J.*, **2**, 27.

Holmes, E. G., Stainer, M. W., Semambo, Y. B. and Jones, E. R. (1951). An investigation of serum proteins of Africans in Uganda. *Trans. roy. Soc. trop. Med. Hyg.*, **45**, 371.

Kibukamusoke, J. W. (1966a). *The Nephrotic Syndrome in Uganda, with special reference to the role of Plasmodium malariae.* M.D. Thesis, University of East Africa. p. 110.

— (1966b). Pyelonephritis as a cause of nephrotic syndrome. *E. Afr. Med. J.*, **43**, 515.

— (1967a). Hypertension and urea retention in proliferative glomerulonephritis. *E. Afr. med. J.*, **44**, 238.

— (1967b). The examination of multiple slides for the demonstration of malaria parasites. *J. trop. Med. Hyg.*, **70**, 46.

Kibukamusoke, J. W., Hutt, M. S. R. and Wilks, N. E. (1967). The nephrotic syndrome in Uganda and its association with quartan malaria. *Quart. J. Med.*, **36**, 393.

— (1968a). Nephrotic syndrome and chronic renal disease in the tropics. *Brit. med. J.*, **2**, 33.

— (1968b). Malaria prophylaxis and immunosuppressant therapy in the management of nephrotic syndrome associated with quartan malaria. *Arch. Dis. Childh.*, **43**, 598.

Lancet (1959). Nephrotic syndrome (leading article). *Lancet*, i, 667.

Lauson, D., Moncrieff, A. and Payne, W. W. (1960). Forty years of nephrosis in childhood. *Arch. Dis. Childh.*, **35**, 115.

Leonard, P. J. and Shaper, A. G. (1965). Serum proteins in African and Asian subjects in Kampala. *E. Afr. med. J.*, **42**, 689.

MacSearraigh, E. T. M., Lewis, M. G., Hutt, M. S. R. and Trussell, R. R. (1969). Cenal biopsy studies in Uganda African women with hypertension in pregnancy. *E. Afr. med. J.*, **46**, 334.

Marsden, P. D., Hutt, M. S. R., Wilks, N. E., Voller, A., Blackman, V., Shah, K. K., Connor, D. H., Hamilton, P. J. S., Banwell, J. G. and Lunn, H. F. (1965). An investigation of tropical splenomegally at Mulago Hospital, Kampala, Uganda. *Brit. med. J.*, **1**, 89.

Ross, J. H. (1960). Recurrent focal nephritis. *Quart. J. Med. (N.S.)*, **29**, 391.

Shaper, A. G. (1968). Immunological studies in a tropical environment. *E. Afr. med. J.*, **45**, 219.

Squire, J. R. (1960). *Functional Pathology. Recent Advances in Renal Disease.* Proceedings of a Conference held at Royal College of Physicians of London. 22–23rd July, 1960. (Edited by Milne, M.D.) pp. 71–89. Pitman, London.

Voller, A. and Bray, R. S. (1962). Fluorescent antibody staining as a measure of malarial antibody. *Proc. Soc. exp. Biol. Med.*, **110**, 907.

White, R. H. R., Glasgow, E. F. and Mills, R. J. (1970). Clinicopathological study of nephrotic syndrome in childhood. *Lancet*, i, 1353.

Wing, A. J., Hutt, M. S. R. and Kibukamusoke, J. W. (1972). Progression and remission in the nephrotic syndrome associated with quartan malaria in Uganda. *Quart. J. Med.*, **41**, 163, 273.

Wilson, S. G. F. and Heymann, W. (1959). Acute glomerulonephritis with the nephrotic syndrome. *Paediatrics*, **23**, 874.

Wing, A. J. (1969). Malignant hypertension with renal failure; a problem in management. *E. Afr. med. J.*, **40**, 321.

3   Biochemical Features

The nephrotic syndrome is defined as a symptom complex comprised of massive proteinuria, hypoalubuminaemia, gross oedema and hypercholestrolaemia (*Lancet*, 1959; Allen, 1962, *British Medical Journal*, 1962). Hardwicke (1954) found that this syndrome appeared when the level of serum albumen was 1·0–2·0 g per cent (25–50 per cent of normal) and that this occurred with a proteinuria of 10–20 g a day in a person weighing 70 kg. Squire (1960) showed that a loss of 7 g per day would be capable of producing the syndrome in people of a smaller build.

In quartan malarial nephropathy the nephrotic syndrome is usually present (Kibukamusoke, Hutt and Wilks, 1967) and often constitutes the initial clinical manifestation of renal involvement in *P. malariae* infections (Chapter 2).

The features given in this chapter are the results of a study of the biochemical changes in 80 consecutive cases of the nephrotic syndrome associated with quartan malaria.

Total plasma proteins

The average plasma protein total was 4·5 g per cent with a range of 2·4–6·6 g per cent. Ten per cent of the cases had values of 3·0 g or below and 4 per cent with values above 5·5 g per cent. The majority (86 per cent) of the cases were therefore in the range of 3·0 to 5·5 g per cent. This is distinctly lower than the average normal for African out-patients (Table 3.1).

Serum albumen

The range was 0·4–2·6 g per cent with an average of 1·2 g per cent. Thirteen per cent of the cases had 0·5 g per cent or below and 6 per cent of the values were above 2 g per cent. These figures are all consistently below the normal (Table 3.1).

Alpha$_2$-globulin

The range was 0·5–1·6 g per cent with only two cases below the normal range of 0·52–0·62 g per cent (Table 3.1). Only 18 per cent of the cases were below 0·7 g per cent. Eighty-two per cent of all the cases, therefore, had values in excess of the normal range.

Table 3·1

Plasma protein levels in different parts of the world

Source	Adults (A) Children (C)	Method	Total protein	Albumen	Alpha₁	Alpha₂	Beta	Gamma
Normal East Africans (Ugandans)								
Holmes et al. (1951)	A	Chemical	7·6	3·27			0·78	1·98
Holmes et al. (1955)	A	Electrophoresis	7·13	3·35			0·67	1·00
Holmes et al. (1955)	C	Electrophoresis	7·16	3·80	0·27	0·62	0·64	1·89
Leonard and Shaper (1965)	A (students)	Electrophoresis	6·82	3·39	0·30	0·56	0·80	1·73
Leonard and Shaper (1965)	A	Electrophoresis	6·74	3·15	0·21	0·52	0·90	1·86
Normal Europeans								
Anderson and Altmann (1951)	A	Electrophoresis	7·2	4·55			0·84	0·95
Holmes et al. (1955)	A	Electrophoresis	6·99	4·59			0·77	0·97
Bayliss (1960)		Electrophoresis	6·3–8·2	4·0–4·5			0·7–1·2	0·7–1·1
Patients with nephrotic syndrome								
Kibukamusoke (present study)	A and C	Electrophoresis	4·5	1·2		0·83	0·83	1·45

Values given in g per cent

Beta-globulin

In slightly more than half of the cases the beta-globulin fraction was present in quantities larger than the alpha$_2$ fraction. The average value for the beta was, however, 0·83 g per cent. These figures are not greater than those given for normal Ugandans (Table 3.1). In fact the highest figure quoted—0·90 g per cent (Leonard and Shaper, 1965) is greater than the average.

Gamma-globulin

This was moderately reduced with an average of 1·45 g per cent as com- pared with the normal range of 1·73–1·98 g per cent (Holmes' figures of 1951 included—Table 3.1). The range was 0·3–4·0 g per cent, 78 per cent with values between 1 and 2 g per cent.

Electrophoretic pattern

Ninety-five per cent of the cases showed the nephrotic pattern—a marked reduction of albumen level, a moderate gamma-globulin reduction and a lone alpha$_2$ or an alpha$_2$-beta pattern (Fig. 3.1) .The remaining 5 per cent

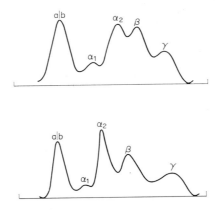

Fig. 3.1. Plasma protein electrophoretic patterns

(a) Case (4N): the alpha$_2$ beta pattern (85 per cent of positive cases)
Total protein: 3·1 g per cent
Albumen: 30 per cent (1·0 g per cent). Alpha$_1$ 10 per cent (0·3 g per cent)
Alpha$_2$: 23 per cent (0·8 g per cent). Beta: 18 per cent (0·5 g per cent)
Gamma: 19 per cent (0·6 g per cent)
(b) Case (66N): Lone alpha$_2$ pattern (10 per cent of the positive cases)
Total protein: 4·0 g per cent
Albumen: 25 per cent (1·0 g per cent). Alpha$_1$: 5 per cent (0·2 g per cent)
Alpha$_2$: 30 per cent (1·3 g per cent). Beta: 24 per cent (1·0 g per cent)
Gamma: 16 per cent (0·5 g per cent)

showed non-diagnostic patterns. Of the positive ones, 85 per cent showed the alpha$_2$-beta pattern—which was therefore the commonest. The rest showed the lone alpha$_2$ pattern.

Serum cholesterol

The range was 140–1,090 mg per cent with only 33 per cent below 300 mg per cent and 12 per cent below 200 mg per cent. Ninety-five per cent were therefore above the normal serum cholesterol level (Shaper and Jones, 1959).

Figure 3.2 shows the relationship between the serum cholesterol level

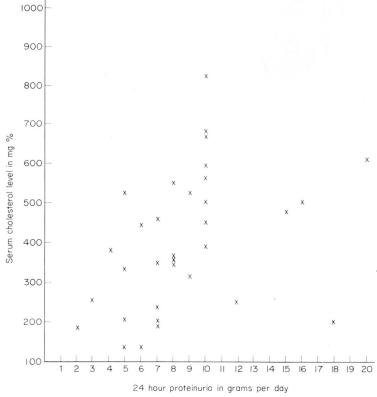

Fig. 3.2. The relationship between serum cholesterol and proteinuria
(Correlation coefficient $(r) = 0.39$; $P < 0.05$)

and the severity of proteinuria. It will be seen that there is a good correlation between the severity of protein loss and the height of the cholesterol level in the blood ($r = 0.39$; $P < 0.05$).

A progressive increase in serum cholesterol level was found to be a fair indication of continued activity of the nephrotic state (Kibukamusoke, 1968).

4

Comment

Thus amidst the considerable confusion that surrounds the subject of oedema in the tropics, it is gratifying to see that relatively simple biochemical tests can serve as an effective means of separating off those cases that are due to the nephrotic syndrome. Serial serum cholesterol estimation was a useful indicator of the activity or otherwise of the nephrotic state. A persistent rise of serum cholesterol very often existed in the presence of active nephrotic syndrome. In these cases too a nephrotic pattern would very often be seen on serum protein electrophoresis. It can therefore be concluded from this work that studies of serum proteins and serum cholesterol are of great value in the diagnosis of the nephrotic syndrome as we see it in Uganda.

BIBLIOGRAPHY

Allen, A. C. (1962). *The Kidney*, (2nd edition). Grune and Stratton, New York.

Anderson, C. G. and Altmann, A. (1951). The electrophoretic serum—protein pattern in malignant malnutrition. *Lancet*, i, 203.

Bayliss, R. I. S. (1960). In *Practical Procedures in Clinical Medicine*. Churchill, London.

British Medical Journal (1962). Leading article. **1**, 383.

Hardwicke, J. (1954). Serum and urinary protein changes in nephrotic syndrome. *Proc. roy. Soc. Med.*, **47**, 832.

Holmes, E. G., Stainer, M. W., Semambo, Y. B. and Jones, E. R. (1951). An investigation of serum proteins of Africans in Uganda. *Trans. roy. Soc. trop. Med. Hyg.*, **45**, 376.

Holmes, E. G., Stainer, M. W. and Thompson, M. D. (1955). The serum protein pattern in Africans in Uganda; relation to diet and malaria. *Trans. roy. Soc. trop. Med. Hyg.*, **49**, 376.

Kibukamusoke, J. W. (1968). Nephrotic syndrome and chronic renal disease in the tropics. *Brit. med. J.*, **2**, 33.

Kibukamusoke, J. W., Hutt, M. S. R. and Wilks, N. E. (1967). Nephrotic syndrome in Uganda and its association with quartan malaria. *Quart. J. Med.*, **36**, 393.

Lancet (1959). Leading article. i, 667.

Leonard, P. J. and Shaper, A. G. (1965). Serum proteins in Africans and Asian subjects in Kampala. *E. Afr. med. J.*, **42**, 689.

Shaper, A. G. and Jones, K. W. (1959). Serum cholesterol, diet, and coronary heart-disease in Africans and Asians in Uganda. *Lancet*, ii, 534.

Squire, J. R. (1960). In *Recent Advances in Renal Diseases*. Proceedings of a Conference held at Royal College of Physicians of London. pp. 71–89. (Edited by Milne, M. D.). Pitman, London.

4 Parasitology

In Chapter 1 a comprehensive review of the knowledge on malarial nephrosis up to the present time was made. In this chapter information on recent work relating to the disease will be discussed. There is today a considerable volume of evidence pointing to *Plasmodium malariae* as a cause of this disease.

World incidence

It is very difficult to find an entirely satisfactory index of the prevalence of a disease in a population particularly if some of the cases resolve spontaneously. However, a simple index derived from the number of new cases admitted to a hospital during the course of one year calculated as a percentage of the total medical admissions gives reproducible results (Kibukamusoke, 1966*b*) (Tables 4.1 and 4.2).

Table 4.1

Percentage of new cases of nephrotic syndrome against total medical admissions in Mulago Hospital, Kampala, Uganda

	1960	1961	1962	1963	1964
New cases of nephrotic syndrome	112	84	105	87	174
Total medical admissions	5,639	5,274	5,727	5,925	6,243
$\dfrac{\text{New cases}}{\text{Total admissions}} \times 100$	2·0	1·6	2·0	1·5	2·8

(After Kibukamusoke, J. W. 1966. The nephrotic syndrome in Uganda with special reference to the role of *Plasmodium malariae*. M.D. Thesis University of East Africa.)

Table 4.2

Year	1963	1964
Total medical admissions	1,119	1,369
Nephrotic syndrome (%)	2·3	2·0

Similar results were obtained from Lagos, Nigeria (Kibukamusoke, 1966*a*) (Table 4.2).

This figure provides a simple and convenient way of comparing the prevalence of the nephrotic syndrome in different parts of the world.

Table 4.3 shows the results of such a survey.

It will be seen from this table that there is a distinct difference between the prevalence of the disease in malarious countries when this is compared with non-malarious countries. In fact the prevalence of the disease is some hundred times greater.

In countries where malaria is coming under effective control the incidence is lower and figures from such areas occupy an intermediate position between the malarious and non-malarious countries.

Effect of rainfall on incidence of the nephrotic syndrome

A curious coincidence of peaks for admissions of cases of the nephrotic syndrome, rainfall and female anopheline mosquito catches (Fig. 4.1) has been reported from Lagos City, Nigeria (Kibukamusoke, 1966*a*). The increase in cases of the nephrotic syndrome in the hospital wards was not due to an increase in total medical admissions to the hospital for these remained at a constantly high level. Nor was it due to a sudden interest in the disease, for the peak in nephrotic admissions appeared in two consecutive years at the same period of the year. The coincidence between the peak of rainfall and nephrotic syndrome could be accounted for by an increase in upper respiratory infections during wet weather as this is a recognised cause of relapse of the nephrotic state, but the recovery of malaria parasites of one particular type from a very large number of the nephrotics could not be explained on this basis. The coincidence between

---

PLATE I

P. malariae

1. Young ring-form trophozoite of quartan malaria. 2, 3, 4. Young trophozoite forms of the parasite showing gradual increase of chromatin and cytoplasm. 5. Developing ring-form trophozoite—elongated chromatin, some pigment apparent. 7, 8, 9, 10, 11, 12. Some forms which the developing trophozoite of quartan may take. 13, 14. Mature trophozites—one a band form. 15, 16, 17, 18, 19. Phases in the development of the schizont (immature schizonts). 20. Mature schizont. 21. Immature microgametocyte. 22. Immature macrogametocyte. 23. Mature microgametocyte. 24. Mature macrogametocyte

PLATE II

P. malariae—thick film

1. Small trophozoites. 2. Growing trophozoites. 3. Mature trophozoites. 4, 5, 6. Immature schizonts with varying numbers of divisions of the chromatin. 7. Mature schizonts. 8. Nucleus of leucocyte. 9. Blood platelets. 10. Cellular remains of young erythrocytes

PLATE I

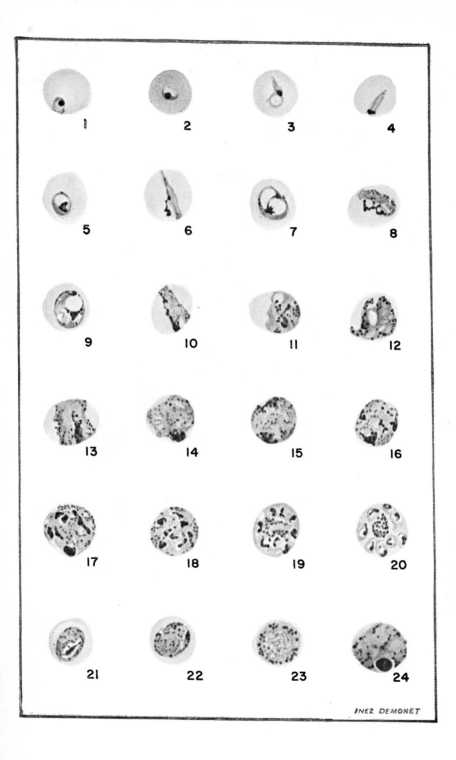

Plate II

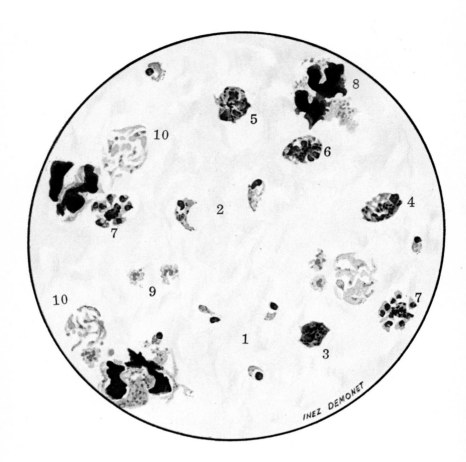

Table 4.3

Incidence of the nephrotic syndrome in different parts of the world

	Country	Hospital	Prevalence of nephrotic syndrome (%)	Malaria status
High incidence	Nigeria	Ibadan*	2·4	Hyperendemic
		Lagos†	2·0	Hyperendemic
	Uganda	Mulago‡	2·0	Hyperendemic
		Fort Portal‡	1·8	Hyperendemic
	Guyana	(British) Guyana (1930)¶	2·8	Pre-malaria eradication
Intermediate incidence	Rhodesia	Salisbury‡	0·67	Effective control
		Bulawayo‡	0·15	Effective control
	Senegal	Dakar§	0·85	Effective control
Low incidence	U.S.A.	California‡	0·03	Complete eradication
		Utah‡	0·15	Complete eradication
	Peoples' Republic of China	Hunan Medical College‡	0·02	Complete eradication
	Guyana (1962)	Demerara¶	0·05	Complete eradication
		Mackenzie Hospital¶	0·05	Complete eradication

* Ikeme, A. C. (1964).
† Kibukamusoke (1966*a*).
‡ Kibukamusoke, Hutt and Wilks (1967).
§ Boisson (1969).
¶ Giglioli (1930) and (1962*a, b*).

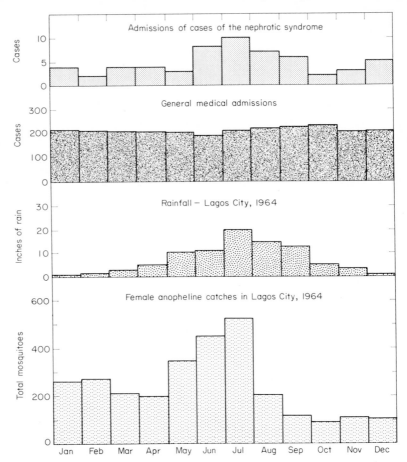

Fig. 4.1. The relationship between monthly rainfall, mosquito density and admissions for the nephrotic syndrome at Lagos University Teaching Hospital (1963 and 1964)

these factors and an agent of malaria transmission thus becomes significant.

Similar studies were done at Mulago Hospital, Kampala (Kibukamusoke, 1971). These studies revealed a 'latent' period of 3 months between the peak incidence of malaria infection and peak admissions for the nephrotic syndrome (Figs. 4.1 and 4.3). It is interesting that Boyd's patients (1940) remained oedema-free for a similar period ($2\frac{1}{2}$ to 3 months). A splenectomised monkey (*A. trivirgatus*) successfully infected with human *P. malariae* at the London School of Hygiene and Tropical Medicine also showed a similar period 17 weeks before nephrotic syndrome developed (Voller *et al.*, 1971). It is therefore to be concluded for the moment that 3 months is the latent period between initial infection and appearance of the nephrotic syndrome.

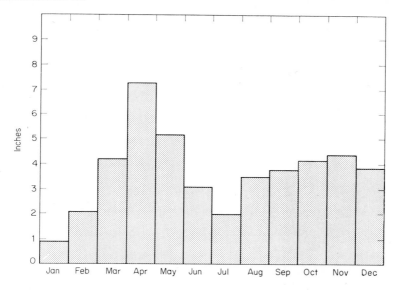

Fig. 4.2. Mean monthly rainfall at Kampala, Uganda

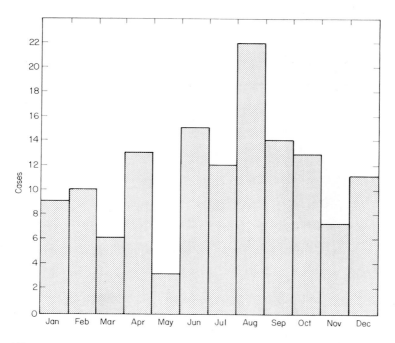

Fig. 4.3. Monthly admissions for the nephrotic syndrome, 1962–1966

Direct studies of malaria parasitaemia

Occurrence of Malaria Parasitaemia in Patients with the Nephrotic Syndrome

Table 4.4 shows the results of a study of nephrotics in age groups 0–10, 10–20 and over 20 years. As might be expected, the youngest patients (0–10 years) show the highest incidence of parasitaemia (80 per cent) and adults have the lowest incidence (40 per cent).

Table 4.4

The incidence of malaria parasitaemia among patients suffering from the nephrotic syndrome

Age in years	Positive cases (%)	Frequency of positive slides in a positive individual
0–10	80	1 in every 1·4
10–20	67	1 in every 3·4
Over 20	40	1 in every 4·5

Children have heavier parasitaemias than adults and consequently give positive slides more frequently than adults.

These figures may simply reflect the parasite density found in different age groups. The last column in Table 4.4 shows a measure of this factor. One in every 1·4 slides were positive for malaria parasites on the multiple slide test (Kibukamusoke, 1967) in children. The frequency of positive slides was least among adults (1 in 4·5) and intermediate in adolescents (1 in 3·4). More direct methods of determining parasite density can also be used (Earle and Perez, 1936). The reasons for these findings will readily be appreciated from Fig. 4.4.

It will be seen from this figure that parasitaemia is progressively suppressed as the malaria antibody titre rises. This occurs as age advances. The multiple slide technique is thus very valuable for the demonstration of the scanty parasitaemia of the adult patient. This is even more necessary in the nephrotic syndrome of quartan malaria where the serum antibodies are even higher (Kibukamusoke, Hutt and Wilks, 1967; Kibukamusoke and Voller, 1970).

The low density of parasitaemias in this disease has already been referred to (Chapter 2). In these cases parasitaemia has also been apparently intermittent. To increase the chances of demonstrating parasitaemia, therefore, one needs to employ special methods. These will now be described.

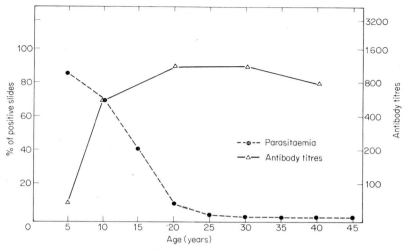

Fig. 4.4. Behaviour of parasitaemia and antibody titres with age

(1) The multiple (serial) slide examination

Useful methods for the demonstration of scanty parasitaemias have been employed by many workers: Bruce-Chwatt, 1963*a*, *b*; Dowling *et al.*, 1966; Kibukamusoke, 1967. The latter described a particularly easy method for this purpose (Kibukamusoke, 1967). In this method a thick blood slide is taken from a drop obtained from a finger prick every day for several days and examined. The entire field of the stained slide is examined under the oil immersion lens. This technique improved parasite recovery rates by two to three times (Table 4.5) (Kibukamusoke, 1967). This was particularly true of *Plasmodium malariae*.

Table 4.5

The effect of multiple (serial) slide examination on demonstration of parasitaemia

		(%)	P. falciparum (%)	P. malariae (%)
Single slide	Population studies (1,810 people)	43	31	4·3
	Non-febrile ward cases (11 patients)	41	41	0·0
Multiple (10) slides	11 (same as above but study continued for 10 days)	71	57	14·0

The incidences are roughly doubled except in cases of *P. malariae* where they are trebled.

Table 4.6

Behaviour of parasitaemia with time (no antimalarials)

Name	Visit 1	2	3	4	5	6	7	8	9	10	11	12	13	14	15	16	17
F.K.	P.M.+	Neg.	Neg.	P.F.+	Neg.	Neg.	Neg.	Neg.	P.F.+	Neg.	Neg.	Neg.	P.F.+	Neg.	Neg.	P.F.+	P.F.+
A.O.	P.F.+	Neg.	Neg.	P.F.+	Neg.	Neg.	Neg.	Neg.	P.F.+								
L.W.	P.F.+	Neg.	Neg.	P.M.+	Neg.	Neg.	P.M.+	Neg.	Neg.	Neg.	Neg.	Neg.	Neg.	Neg.	Neg.		
N.S.	Neg.	Neg.	P.F.+	Neg.	Neg.	Neg.											
M.K.	Neg.	Neg.	P.F.+	Neg.	P.F.+	P.F.+											

10 Thick slides were examined at each session.
No antimalarials were given prior to the blood slide examinations.

Throughout all this period the patient should be sheltered from further infection as this might interfere with the results. At Mulago this was ensured by admission to hospital where no malaria transmission occurs.

It is equally important to avoid all antimalarials as even a minute dose may abolish a parasitaemia that is scanty.

(2) The multiple (sessional) slide examination

The chances of demonstrating a light parasitaemia might be increased by the examination of several slides taken at one sitting. Kibukamusoke (1967) described a suitable method in which he took five to ten thick slides at each session. This method was suitable for out-patients at each clinic visit. It was also convenient for in-patients as it avoided the difficulties of a 10-day study (multiple (serial) slide examination). Using this method a clear pattern appeared to emerge: either all the slides were negative or several were positive (Tables 4.6 and 4.7). The results seemed to suggest that parasitaemia was present only on particular occasions (intermittently). This parasitaemia could, however, have been missed if only one slide had been taken. In Case 8 (J.O.) (Table 4.7), for instance, only 3 out of 10 slides showed malaria parasites and these were few in number. Whilst it is difficult to state how much this method improves the chances of detecting a light parasitaemia its usefulness is obvious. It is the method the author now employs routinely.

(3) Four-hourly blood slide examination

An attempt was made to find out whether a study of blood slides taken every four hours throughout the cycle of 72 hours provided any advantages over the two methods described above.

Twenty-three cases were studied in this way and only two (patients A and B) were positive for malaria parasites (Tables 4.8 and 4.9).

In patient A (a child of 6) parasites would have been found in a single slide as the parasite density was relatively high. Parasitaemia was continuously present throughout the 72-hour period. This was true for *P. malariae* but *P. falciparum* was found in only 3 slides taken at 4 a.m., 12 m.d. and 4 p.m. It is therefore impossible to suggest a particular time when one could have been able to demonstrate *P. falciparum* in this case.

Patient B (another child of 12) only showed parasites in 3 slides taken at 6 p.m., 10 a.m., and 2 a.m. Parasite density was very low. Again it would have been impossible to know when one would have the greatest chance of finding parasites. It is possible, however, that 10 slides taken at one sitting could have shown parasites in some of them. As the 4-hourly method has not demonstrated any outstanding advantages it is not recommended.

Table 4.7

Results on multiple slides taken at each visit—
sessional multiple slide studies

No.	Name	1st visit	2nd visit	3rd visit	Comment
1	N.	10 Neg.	10 Neg.	5 P.F.	
2	O.	10 Neg.	—	5 Neg.	Previously P.M. +ve primaquine/ chloroquine course given 2/12 previously
3	J.S.	5 Neg.	10 Neg.	—	
4	F.S.	5 Neg.	5 Neg.	—	
5	R.N.	5 Neg.	2 +ve P.M. 3 Neg.	5 Neg.	Attacks of fever suggestive of malaria two weeks previous to second visit
6	B.	5 Neg.	—	—	Mild fever due to sore throat
7	N.	10 Neg.	5 Neg.	—	
8	J.O.	5 Neg.	3 +ve P.M. 7 Neg.	10 Neg.	Evening fevers prior to second visit; spleen 4 fb
9	A.K.	5 Neg.	10 Neg.	—	Previously positive for P.M. No antimalarials given
10	S.	10 Neg.	—	—	
11	S.M.	10 Neg.	5 Neg.	5 Neg.	
12	J.M.	5 Neg.	5 Neg.	—	Previously +ve for P.M. No treatment given
13	E.B.	5 Neg.	—	—	
14	M.M.	5 +ve P.M. 5 Neg.	5 Neg.	5 Neg.	
15	S.B.	5 Neg.	10 Neg.	—	
16	S.T.	5 Neg.	10 Neg.	5 P.F.	
17	W.	5 Neg.	—	—	
18	W.L.	5 Neg.	10 Neg.	5 Neg.	
19	P.D.	5 Neg.	—	—	

None of the patients was receiving antimalarials and all were normally exposed to hyperendemic malaria.
The intermittent nature of parasitaemia is clearly demonstrated.
P.M. = *Plasmodium malariae*. P.F. = *Plasmodium falciparum*.

Table 4.8

Patient A

25.11.67	16.00 hr	P.M.		27.11.67	04.00 hr	P.M.
	20.00 hr	P.M.			08.00 hr	P.M.
	00.00 hr	P.M.			12.00 hr	P.F. + P.M.
26.11.67	04.00 hr	P.F. + P.M.			16.00 hr	P.M.
	08.00 hr	P.M.			20.00 hr	P.M.
	12.00 hr	P.M.		28.11.67	00.00 hr	P.M.
	16.00 hr	P.M.			04.00 hr	P.M.
	20.00 hr	P.M.			08.00 hr	P.M.
	00.00 hr	P.M.			12.00 hr	P.M.
					16.00 hr	P.F. + P.M.

P.F. = *Plasmodium falciparum*. P.M. = *Plasmodium malariae*.

Table 4.9

Patient B

13.7.67	14.00 hr	Neg.			06.00 hr	Neg.
	18.00 hr	P.F.			10.00 hr	Neg.
	22.00 hr	Neg.			14.00 hr	Neg.
14.7.67	02.00 hr	Neg.			18.00 hr	Neg.
	06.00 hr	Neg.			22.00 hr	Neg.
	10.00 hr	P.F.		16.7.67	02.00 hr	P.F.
	14.00 hr	Neg.			06.00 hr	Neg.
	18.00 hr	Neg.			10.00 hr	Neg.
	22.00 hr	Neg.			14.00 hr	Neg.
15.7.67	02.00 hr	Neg.				

P.F. = *P. falciparum.*
Only three slides were positive for malaria parasites.

In the rest of the 21 cases a scanty parasitaemia was found subsequently in 3 cases (after 8, 11 and 14 days) by the multiple sessional slide method (with 10 thick slides at a sitting).

The best time to take slides is when a slight temperature (say 99° F, 37·2° C) is detected on the temperature chart or when symptoms of vague ill-health (in an immune person), e.g. anorexia or lassitude, are complained of.

'Intermittent' appearance of parasitaemia

Opinion is divided on the question of whether malaria parasites can be truly absent from the circulation during periods of remission or latency. The hypothesis of relapses appears to be based on only two observations in monkeys (Shortt and Garnham, 1948*b*; Shortt, Bray and Cooper, 1954). These workers demonstrated the presence of exo-erythrocytic forms of *P. cynomolgi* in the animals' liver. Unfortunately many others have failed to do so even in cases where the probability of finding these forms was high. Corradetti and Verolini (1951) were unable to repeat these findings in 4 monkeys infected with sporozoites of *P. cynomolgi* despite careful examination of many hundreds of sections from the livers. One of the animals was sacrificed on the first day of a long-term relapse of parasitae-mia—a situation in which the liver forms would be expected to be found—but none were discovered on examination of numerous sections from the liver. It is also to be expected that the persistence of liver forms would be due to invasion of fresh neighbouring liver cells by merozoites form a ruptured schizont. Shortt and Garnham (1948*a*) were unable to demon-strate this but showed that apart from entering the blood stream, the merozoites were rapidly phagocytosed by macrophages which invade the hepatic area harbouring the schizont.

Golgi (1893) considered that relapses of parasitaemia were due to the revival of malaria parasites engulfed by phagocytes and in this way protected from other injuring agents. Bignami (1910), however, felt that relapses could be due to the survival of minimal numbers of parasites in the circulation for these could occasionally be revealed by accurate microscopy during periods of latency. Corradetti (1966) also felt that this was possible but that the parasites probably survived in secluded capillaries of the internal organs and that these would revive and invade the general circulation when host conditions for their growth and multiplication appeared. Such conditions might be present after splenectomy.

The occurrence of prolonged relapses in plasmodial infections known not to have a persisting liver form such as *P. falciparum* would favour this explanation. Numerous reports have appeared confirming this: Eyles and Young (1951) 480 days; Logan (1953) 4 years; Jeffery and Eyles (1954) 503 days; Ciuca *et al.* (1955) 27 months; Walters (1960) 19 months; Russell *et al.* (1963) 4 years; Verdrager (1964) 3 years. All these patients enjoyed long remissions from malaria parasitaemia. If this is possible with *P. falciparum* it might also be conceivably possible with other human plasmodia.

The failure to infect a susceptible host with blood from patients in remission on many occasions is, however, against this theory. Corradetti himself experienced this failure when he was unable to infect a susceptible host under these circumstances (Corradetti and Verolini, 1951).

Fairley (1945), Copper *et al.* (1949) and Coatney *et al.* (1950) also had similar experiences. This does not completely rule out the possibility of 'parasite hibernation' referred to above but suggests that it is unlikely.

The possibility of total aparasitaemia is more probable in some of our cases who experienced prolonged remissions (Fig. 4.5). It may also provide an explanation for the apparent benefit we previously reported with prolonged malaria prophylaxis (Kibukamusoke, 1968).

The appearance of parasites has so often been associated with an increase in malaria antibody titres (Fig. 4.5) that the repeated finding of low antibody titres (Fig. 4.5) strongly suggests that the failure to find parasites in several blood slides taken on each occasion indicates a state of true aparasitaemia.

Coincidence of the peak incidence of the nephrotic syndrome in children with peak malaria infection

In 1963 Gilles and Hendrickse reported that *P. malariae* infection reached its maximum intensity between the ages of 3 and 7 years in the village communities near Ibadan and that it virtually faded out in adult life to an incidence of 2–3 per cent. These workers also found that the age distribution of the admissions for nephrotic syndrome in children showed a similar curve—reaching a peak between the ages of 5 and 7 years. A comparison between the ages at onset of the nephrotic syndrome in Nigerian and American children showed that the peak for the former was shifted and curiously coincided with peak malaria infection.

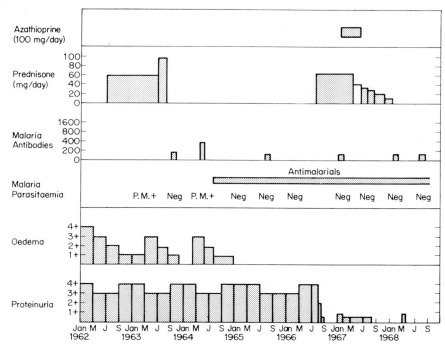

Fig. 4.5. The nephrotic syndrome associated with quartan malaria

Clinical record: L.W. aged 15, male

Proteinuria reduced to a trace by steroids after prolonged malaria prophylaxis, this was then abolished by azathioprine

P. malariae infections were associated with episodes of oedema and increase of malaria antibodies

Kibukamusoke and his associates (1967) reported similar findings (Fig. 4.6).

These observations suggest that the shift is due to malaria and that it is probably caused by it.

Reversal of Plasmodium falciparum : malariae ratio

In East Africa as indeed in most of the heavily malarious countries the common causative agent is *Plasmodium falciparum* and this parasite is found in most of the slides positive for malaria. *P. malariae* is next in frequency and often accounts for 30 per cent of the positive slides for malaria in some areas. The *falciparum:malariae* ratio (P.F.:P.M.) is therefore always 2:1 or higher. In some areas this ratio reaches 5:1 and rarely 5:0; when *P. malariae* appears to be completely absent.

These relationships are shown in Table 4.10 which is derived from a study in Kampala.

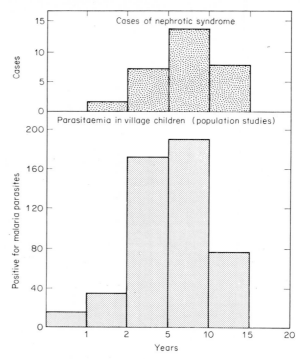

Fig. 4.6. Coincidence of the peak incidence of nephrotic syndrome
with peak malaria infection in children

Table 4.10

*Parasite rates among controls and patients with the
nephrotic syndrome in Uganda*

Age	Cases (%)	Controls (Single slide examinations)			
		Hospital patients (%)	Inhabitants of 3 villages		
			(a) (%)	(b) (%)	(c) (%)
Children (0–14 yr)	81 (1:5)	16 (5:1)	12 (2½:1)	22 (4:1)	23 (2:1)
Adults (Over 20 yr)	40 (2:3)	17 (1:1)	10 (4:1)	6 (5:0)	6 (3:1)

P.F.:P.M. ratio is given in brackets. It is reversed in cases of the nephrotic syndrome.

It will be noticed that the P.F.:P.M. ratio is reversed in cases suffering
from the nephrotic syndrome. This means that there is a relatively greater
frequency of *Plasmodium malariae* in cases of the nephrotic syndrome.

This frequency is confirmed when carefully matched control subjects are studied along with cases of the nephrotic syndrome (Table 4.11).

Table 4.11

Malaria parasitaemia in patients with the nephrotic syndrome and matched controls

Age group	Subjects	Total number	Patients showing Plasmodia		Mixed P.F./ P.M.	Incidence of parasit- aemia in group
			malariae	*falciparum*		
Children (0–14)	Patients	16	9	3	1	13/16
	Matched controls	16	1	2	—	3/16
Adults (18 and over)	Patients	21	3	2	—	5/21
	Matched controls	21	1	2	—	3/21

The rate of parasitaemia is significantly different between childhood patients and their controls ($P < 0.01$). This difference is due to a selective increase in *Plasmodium malariae* parasitaemia.

Incidence of the different plasmodial species in patients and matched controls

The multiple serial slide technique (Kibukamusoke, 1967) was used to study parasitaemia in 16 children suffering from the nephrotic syndrome at Mulago and 21 adults. Each patient was carefully matched with a control for age, sex, tribe and period of exposure to hyperendemic malaria. The results are presented in Table 4.11.

The chi-squared test (χ^2) on these figures reveals that the frequency of *Plasmodium malariae* is significantly greater among children suffering from the nephrotic syndrome than among matched controls ($P < 0.01$). There is also a significantly greater incidence of (total) malaria parasitaemia among childhood cases than among their controls ($P < 0.02$). The frequency of *Plasmodium falciparum* in both groups, however, is not different. *Plasmodium malariae* therefore shows a selective increase in cases of the nephrotic syndrome and solely contributes to the overall increase of malaria parasitaemia in this group.

The position is different with the adults. This test shows no statistical difference either in the frequency of *Plasmodium malariae* among the adult cases of nephrotic syndrome nor in the overall incidence of parasitaemia in this group. The most likely reason for this observation is parasite suppression from antibodies in the malarial immune state (Fig. 4.4). Cohen and McGregor (1963) demonstrated antiplasmodial effect of 7S gamma globulin and later McGregor (1964) showed its parasiticidal effect on the asexual (erythrocytic form) parasite. It is therefore unwise to interpret this finding to mean non-association with *Plasmodium malariae*. Further evidence incriminating this parasite will be given in Chapter 6.

The nephrotic syndrome has now been successfully produced in *Aotus trivirgatus* at the London School of Hygiene and Tropical Medicine. This monkey was splenectomised and infected with *P. malariae* (of human origin) in December 1970. The monkey developed nephrotic syndrome during a second relapse of parasitaemia. Immunofluorescent staining of frozen renal tissue demonstrated a granular deposit composed of IgM and no IgG at all. Optical microscopy showed a membrano-proliferative glomerulonephritis of moderate severity. (Voller *et al.* (1971).)

Possible role of other human plasmodia

P. vivax was used for many years in pyrexial therapy of the nephrotic syndrome. Accounts of these patients, however, do not suggest any possible aggravation of the disease in any of them. On the contrary a number showed improvement in the general clinical state particularly with reference to oedema.

The occurrence of proteinuria in uncomplicated *P. falciparum* infections is well known but the incidence of proteinuria is higher in *P. malariae* infections (Giglioli, 1930)—Table 2.1.

Berger, Birch and Conte (1967) reported three patients with *falciparum* malaria who developed features of renal involvement. The data they give, however, are not in full agreement with a diagnosis of the nephrotic syndrome as classically described (*Lancet*, 1959), nor are they comparable with typical cases of the nephrotic syndrome of quartan malaria (Kibuka-musoke, Hutt and Wilks, 1967). The figures, however, indicate that glomerulonephritis was present.

P. vivax was present in some of Giglioli's patients but the weight of the evidence was against this parasite as a cause of renal disease (Giglioli, 1930). In British Guyana, where this author worked, *P. vivax* was very prevalent and this appears to explain the frequency of this parasite in the series. Thus the presence of *P. vivax* in Giglioli's series seemed to be fortuitous.

P. falciparum on the other hand was extremely rarely found in these patients and when it did appear it was in association with *P. vivax*.

P. falciparum, however, was apparently responsible for some of the relapses in a small number of my cases (Fig. 7.1) though in many others fresh infections with this parasite did not appear to be followed by a relapse (Fig. 4.7). A possible reason for this is discussed in Chapter 6.

The role of *P. malariae* in the syndrome

Evidence has now been given of a relationship between *Plasmodium malariae* and the nephrotic syndrome, and it is now appropriate to consider the role this parasite plays in the disease. In theory it could be a question

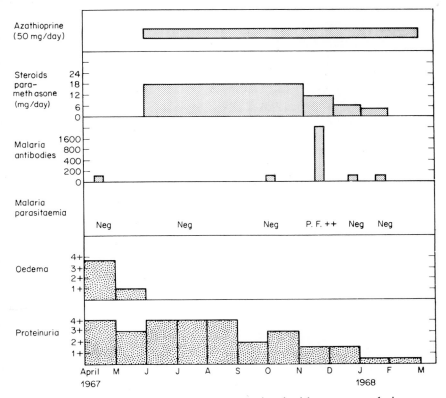

Fig. 4.7. The nephrotic syndrome associated with quartan malaria

Clinical record: S.N., aged 13, male

A fresh infection with *P. falciparum* did not produce a recurrence of oedema or proteinuria though it was associated with a considerable rise in malaria antibodies

of seed or soil. This means that the presence of *P. malariae* in these cases may reflect an undue susceptibility to this parasite or alternatively that the parasite causes the disease.

Four main pieces of evidence suggest that the parasite is involved in the causation of the disease:

(1) The most direct evidence is derived from the work of Boyd (1940) who administered *P. malariae* to psychiatric patients for therapeutic purposes and observed that a number of them developed what is now recognised as the nephrotic syndrome. He reported, however, that proteinuria disappeared after termination of the infection by quinine. This is contrary to our experiences and the answer may well be in the state of immunity towards malaria prior to the fateful infection. The work of Voller *et al.* (1971) also suggests a direct causal relationship.

(2) Giglioli (1962*a*, *b*) reviewed the situation in Guyana following the introduction of malaria control. He found that a concurrent reduction in

the incidence of both the nephrotic syndrome and chronic renal disease had taken place. If the occurrence of *P. malariae* in the *nephrotic syndrome* was merely because of increased susceptibility then the only expected change would be a reduction in the numbers of cases of the syndrome from whom parasites were recoverable. A concurrent decrease in the numbers of the nephrotic syndrome therefore suggests a direct causal relationship— a removal of the causative agent. It is possible of course that another factor was removed at the same time, but this is rather unlikely.

(3) Allison and his associates (1969) in a careful investigation using eluates from the kidney of a child who died of this syndrome and showing granular immune deposits by electron and fluorescence microscopy obtained a precipitate with an extract of the spleen from the same patient. This spleen was shown to contain *P. malariae* parasites. No precipitate was obtained with the spleen of another child containing *P. falciparum* parasites; nor did a cryostat section of normal kidney show fluorescence with the labelled eluted antibody. This indicated that there was a specific *P. malariae* antigen present in the kidney of patients with this condition which was absent in *P. falciparum* infection. The finding of soluble complexes in the same kidney suggests that the *P. malariae* antigen is concerned directly with their formation and consequently with the damage they cause.

(4) The shift of the peak incidence of nephrotic syndrome from the age of two as seen in the temperate climate (Barnett *et al.*, 1952) to coincide with peak malaria infection at the age of 5–7 years also strongly supports the hypothesis of cause and effect.

Nephropathy in simian malaria

This is a greatly neglected field despite extensive work with simian plasmodia. It is clear that many of the puzzling problems in the nephrotic syndrome of quartan malaria will lend themselves to investigation and study through work with experimental infections in laboratory animals.

Desowitz *et al.* (1968) and Ward (1966) have attempted to investigate this field. Desowitz and his associates were interested in the pathology and host physiology of a variety of simian plasmodia. One of their studies concerned the patho-physiology of *Plasmodium inui* infections. This parasite is interesting because it is a potential model for human *P. malariae*. *P. inui* resembles the human quartan malaria parasite in its morphology and schizogonic behaviour.

As in *P. coatneyi* malaria Desowitz *et al.* (1968) found a wide variation in the intensity of *P. inui* infection. These workers also found (as expected) that anaemias and parasitaemias were severer in the splenectomised monkeys. Two of their monkeys showed renal involvement after 200 days of infection in one monkey and 174 in the other. Both monkeys showed serious damage to the kidneys. The urine showed corresponding changes: red cell and granular casts, heavy proteinuria and large numbers of white cells. There was a progressive rise in blood urea nitrogen and creatinine. One of the monkeys died. Its kidney showed an acute proliferative glomerulonephritis and this progressed to extensive obliteration of glomerular tufts with prominent epithelial crescents. This feature of epithelial crescents is, however, unknown in typical human quartan malaria nephropathy. In addition abundant haemozoin occurred in the damaged glomeruli, contrary to human cases.

The second monkey survived and after the attack no further evidence of renal involvement was found except that a renal biopsy taken a year later revealed focal obliterative glomerulitis involving two of the ten glomeruli seen in the sections. The renal biopsies on all the rest of the (5) monkeys between days 110 and 470 showed entirely normal histologies, though haemozoin was present in the glomeruli in all instances.

Ward and Conran (1966) were interested in studying the immunological changes in various tissues in malaria particularly as it had been demonstrated by Weigle (1964) and Dixon (1963) that soluble immune complexes could cause a local increase in vascular permeability, generalised anaphylaxis, acute vasculitis and glomerulonephritis.

Using blood infections of *Plasmodium cynomolgi* in splenectomised Rhesus monkeys they studied fluorescent stained sections of liver and kidney. In addition to antigenic breakdown products in the reticuloendo-thelial system of the liver, these workers found focal deposits of malaria antigenic material in renal capillary loops. The pattern of fluorescence was linear and visible along capillary endothelial surfaces. Linear subendothelial deposits, however, are not typical of immune complex disease. Associated with these deposits of malaria antigenic material monkey gammaglobulin and βIC-globulin was detected. The deposits in the kidney were found only in monkeys which had been ill for two or three weeks with malaria, suggesting an immunological event. Further studies by these workers (Ward and Conran, 1969) has been summarised in Chapter 6.

Sesta *et al.* (1968) studied the renal lesion which occurs in the golden hamster in *Plasmodium berghei* infections. This, however, was an acute tubular necrosis type of lesion similar to the renal lesion of *P. knowlesi* in Rhesus monkeys (Rosen *et al.*, 1968) and *P. falciparum* in man (Maegraith, 1948). It is unlike the glomerular lesions of *P. inui* or *P. cynomolgi* in monkeys.

One of the main problems in this field has been the failure to infect laboratory animals with human plasmodia. It is encouraging to note that this difficulty is now being overcome. Rodhain (1948) was the first person to report that it was possible to infect young chimpanzees with *P. malariae* and Garnham *et al.* (1956) studied the behaviour of this parasite in a splenectomised chimpanzee. Bray (1960) continued this work and fed *Anopheles gambiae* on human beings and on chimpanzees infected with *P. malariae* on 38 occasions. The mosquitoes became infected in many cases and in a number of instances he was able to transmit the *P. malariae* infections from man to the chimpanzees.

In 1966, Young, Porter and Johnson reported a successful transmission of human plasmodia to animals. These workers successfully infected a New World monkey (*Aotus trivirgatus*—owl monkey) with *P. vivax* and subsequently got it back into a human being. This work was soon confirmed by Geiman and Meagher (1967) who used the same monkey for a *P. falciparum* infection from a human subject. They maintained the infection by serial passage. Geiman and Siddiqui (1969) reported the successful infection of the same monkey with *P. malariae* from a congenital case aged 8 weeks. These workers were able to show that infections with this parasite can be maintained for a year or more and that they can be passed to non-splenectomised *Aotus*.

Infection of *Aotus trivirgatus* with *P. malariae* has thus opened new possibilities in the field of research on quartan malarial nephropathy. The infection is characterised by a long prepatent period and a low level of parasitaemia extended for a long period of time. So far the indications are that *P. malariae* in *A. trivirgatus* produces similar morphological asexual forms, levels of parasitaemia and duration of infection as it does in man (Geiman and Siddiqui, 1969). Several other workers have now achieved the same success (Contacos and Collins, 1969; Voller *et al.*, 1971; Wilks, 1969).

BIBLIOGRAPHY

Allison, A. C., Houba, V., Hendrickse, R. G., de Petris, S., Edington, G. M. and Adeniyi, A. (1969). Immune complexes in the nephrotic syndrome in African children. *Lancet*, i, 1232.

Barnett, H. L., Forman, C. W. and Lauson, H. D. (1952). The nephrotic syndrome in children. *Adv. Paediat.*, **5**, 53.

Berger, M., Birch, L. M. and Conte, N. F. (1967). The nephrotic syndrome secondary to acute glomerulonephritis during falciparum malaria. *Ann. Int. Med.* 67, **6**, 1163.

Bignami, A. (1910). Sulla petogenosi delle recidive nelle febri Malariche. *Att. Soc. Stud. Malaria*, **11**, 731.

Boisson, Marie-Eglantine (1969). *Étude anatomo-clinique du syndrome nephrotique chez l'enfant noir aux Senegal*. M.D. Thesis, Faculté de Médécine de Montpellier.

Boyd, M. F. (1940). Observations on naturally and artificially induced quartan malaria. *Amer. J. trop. Med.*, **20**, 749.

Bray, R. S. (1960). Studies on malaria in chimpanzees. VIII. The experimental transmission and pre-erythrocytic phase of *Plasmodium malariae*, with a note on the host range of the parasite. *Amer J. trop. Med. Hyg.*, **9**, 455.

Bruce-Chwatt, L. J. (1963a). A longitudinal survey of natural malaria infection in a group of West African adults. *W. Afr. med. J.*, **12**, 141.

— (1963b). A longitudinal survey of natural malaria infection in group of West African adults. *W. Afr. med. J.*, **12**, 199.

Ciuca, M., *et al.* (1955). *Bull Sti. Sec. St. Med. (Bucharest)*, **7**, 61.

Coatney, G. R., Cooper, W. C. and Ruhe, D. S. (1947). Studies in human malaria. V. Homologons strain superinfection during latency in subjects with sporozoite-induced *vivax* malaria (St. Elizabeth strain). *Amer. J. Hyg.*, **46**, 141.

Coatney, G. R., Cooper, W. C. and Young, M. D. (1950). Studies of human malaria; summary of 204 sporozoite-induced infections with chesson strain of *Plasmodium vivax*. *J. nat. Malaria Soc.*, **9**, 381.

Cohen, S. and McGregor, I. A. (1963). In *Immunity to Protozoa*. (Edited by Garnham P. C. C., Pierce, A. E. and Roitt, I.) Blackwell, Oxford.

Contacos, P. G. and Collins, W. E. (1969). Transmission from monkey to man by mosquito bite. *Science*, **165**, 918.

Cooper, W. C., Ruhe, D. S. and Coatney, G. R. (1949). Studies in human malaria. XVI. Results of massive subinoculation during latency from patients infected with St. Elizabeth strain, *vivax* malaria. *Amer. J. Hyg.*, **50**, 189.

Corradetti, A. and Verolini, F. (1951). Studie Sulle recidive da *P. malariae* e da *P. cynomolgi* in infezioni indotte con sangue, R. C. 1st suppl. *Sanita*, **14**, 271.

Corradetti, A. (1966). The origin of relapses in human and simian malaria infections. WHO/Mal./**66**, 565.

Desowitz, R. S., Miller, L. H., Buchanan, R. D. and Permanich, B. (1968). Comparative studies on the pathology and host physiology of malarias. *Plasmodium inui*. *Ann. trop. Med. Parasit.*, **62**, 233.

Dixon, F. J. (1963). *Harvey Lect.*. **58**, 21.

Dowling, M. A. C., Richman, L. R., Shute, G. T. and Menzies, M. G. F. (1966). A field method of blood concentration for improved diagnosis of scanty parasitaemia, in Malaria practice. WHO/Mal./**66**, 535.

Earle, W. S. and Perez, M. (1936). Enumeration of parasites in the blood of malarial patients. *J. Lab. clin. Med.*, **17**, 1124.

Eyles, D. E. and Young, M. D. (1951). Duration of untreated and inadequately treated *Plasmodium falciparum* infections in human host. *J. nat. Malaria Soc.*, **10**, 327.

Fairley, N. H. (1945). Chemotherapeutic suppression and prophylaxis in malaria; an experimental investigation undertaken by medical research teams in Australia. *Trans. roy. Soc. trop. Med. Hyg.*, **38**, 311.

Garnham, P. C. C., Lauson, R. and Gunders, A. E. (1956). Some observations on malaria parasites in a chimpanzee with particular reference to the persistence of *Plasmodium reichenowi* and *Plasmodium vivax*. *Ann. Soc. belge Méd. trop.*, **36**, 811.

Geiman, Q. M. and Meagher, M. J. (1967). Susceptibility of a New World monkey to *Plasmodium falciparum* from man. *Nature* (Lond.), **215**, 437.

Geiman, Q. M. and Siddiqui, W. A. (1969). Susceptibility of a New World monkey to *Plasmodium falciparum* from man. *Amer. J. trop. Med. Hyg.*, **18**, 351.

Giglioli, G. (1930). *Malarial Nephritis*. Churchill, London.

Giglioli, G. (1962a). Malaria and renal disease, with special reference to British Guiana. I. Introduction. *Ann. trop. Med. Parasit.*, **56**, 101.

Giglioli, G. (1962b). Malaria and renal disease, with special reference to British Guiana. II. The effect of malaria eradication on the incidence of renal disease in British Guiana. *Ann. trop. Med. Parasit.*, **56**, 225.

Gilles, H. M. and Hendrickse, R. G. (1963). Nephrosis in Nigerian children; role of *Plasmodium malaride*, and effect of antimalarial treatment. *Brit. med. J.*, **2**, 27.

Golgi, C. (1893). Sulle felori malariche estivo antunnali di Roma. *Gazz. med. Pavia*, 2 Nov. Die. (Reprinted in: Gli studi di canillo Golgi Sulla Malaria raccotti e ordinati da A. Perroneito, Rome 1929).

Ikeme, A. C. (1964). Personal communication.

Jeffery, G. M. and Eyles, D. E. (1954). Duration in human host of infections with Panama strain of *Plasmodium falciparum*. *Amer. J. trop. Med. Hyg.*, **3**, 219.

Kibukamusoke, J. W. (1966a). The nephrotic syndrome in Lagos, Nigeria. *W. Afr. med. J.*, **15**, 213.

— (1966b). *The nephrotic syndrome in Uganda with special reference to the role of Plasmodium malariae*. M.D. Thesis, University of East Africa.

— (1967). The examination of multiple slides for the demonstration of malaria parasites. *J. trop. Med. Hyg.*, **70**, 46.

Kibukamusoke, J. W. (1968). Malaria prophylaxis and immunosuppressant therapy in the management of nephrotic syndrome associated with quartan malaria. *Arch Dis. Childh.*, **48**, 598.

— (1971). Rainfall and admissions for the nephrotic syndrome. *E. Afr. med. J.*, **48**, 13.

Kibukamusoke, J. W., Hutt, M. S. R. and Wilks, N. E. (1967). The nephrotic syndrome in Uganda and its association with quartan malaria. *Quart. J. Med.*, **36**, 393.

Kibukamusoke, J. W. and Voller, A. (1970). Serological studies on nephrotic syndrome of quartan malaria in Uganda. *Brit. med. J.*, **1**, 406.

Lancet (1959). Nephrotic syndrome. Leading article. i, 667.

Logan, J. A. (1953). *The Sardinian Project, Baltimore.* Johns Hopkins, Baltimore.

McGregor, I. A. (1964). The passive transfer of human malarial immunity. *Amer. J. trop. Med. Hyg.*, **13**, 237.

Maegraith, B. G. (1948). *Pathological Processes in Malaria and Blackwater Fever* Blackwell, Oxford.

Rodhain, J. (1948). Susceptibility of chimpanzee to *Plasmodium malariae* of human origin. *Amer. J. trop. Med.*, **28**, 629.

Rosen, S., Hano, J. E. and Barry, K. G. (1968). Malarial nephropathy in the Rhesus monkey. *Arch. Path.*, **85**, 36.

Russell, P. E., West, L. S., Hanwell, R. D. and MacDonald, G. (1963). In *Practical Malariology*. Oxford University Press, London.

Sesta, J. J., Rosen, S. and Sprinz, H. (1968). Malarial nephropathy in the golden hamster. *Arch. Path.*, **85**, 644.

Shortt, H. E., Bray, R. S. and Cooper, W. (1954). Further notes on the tissue stages of *Plasmodium cynomolgi. Trans. roy. Soc. trop. Med. Hyg.*, **48**, 122.

Shortt, H. E. and Garnham, P. C. C. (1948a). The pre-erythrocytic development of *Plasmodium cynomolgi* and *Plasmodium vivax. Trans. roy. Soc. trop. Med. Hyg.*, **41**, 785.

— (1948b). Demonstration of a persisting exo-erythrocytic cycle in *Plasmodium cynomolgi* and its bearing on the production of relapses. *Brit. med. J.*, **1**, 1225.

Verdrager, J. (1964). Observations on the longevity of *Plasmodium falciparum.* WHO/Mal./431.

Voller, A., Draper, C. C., Shwe T. and Hutt, M. S. R. (1971). *Brit. med. J.*, **4**, 208.

Walters, J. (1960). Quiescent malarial parasites. *Brit. med. J.*, **1**, 1206.

Ward, P. A. and Conran, P. B. (1966). Immuno-pathologic studies of simian malaria. *Milit. Med.*, **131**, No. 9 Supplement, 1225.

— (1969). Immunopathology of renal complications in simian malaria and human quartan malaria. *Milit. Med.*, **134**, 10, 1228.

Weigle, W. O. (1964). Mechanisms of antibody formation. *Advanc. Immunol.*, **1**, 283.

Wilks, N. E. (1969). Personal communication.

Young, M. D., Porter, J. A. and Johnson, C. M. (1966). *Plasmodium vivax* transmitted from man to monkey to man. *Science*, **153**, 1006.

5 Pathology

The nephrotic syndrome develops when there are widespread persistent abnormalities of the glomeruli which result in gross proteinuria with subsequent hypoproteinaemia.

The syndrome may be associated with systemic diseases which involve the glomeruli by a variety of pathogenetic mechanisms: Amyloidosis, the glomerular lesions of diabetes mellitus, renal vein thrombosis and renal involvement in diseases such as disseminated lupus erythematosus are examples of conditions where there are specific extra-renal findings. The great majority of cases, however, are due to primary glomerular disease, unassociated with systemic lesions. In strict pathological terms glomerulonephritis should be reserved for lesions which have characteristics of inflammation, such as proliferation. However, the term is often extended to include other types of primary glomerular disease and is used in this wider sense in this chapter.

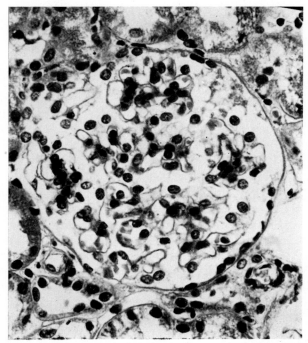

Fig. 5.1. Minimal change. The glomerulus is normal apart from a possible increase in mesangial nuclei. H and E. × 480

Cases with the nephrotic syndrome due to glomerulonephritis can be divided into three main categories on histological grounds. These are: minimal (nil) lesion, membranous glomerulonephritis (membranous nephropathy) and proliferative glomerulonephritis. As the term suggests the glomeruli in minimal change cases show little or no abnormality on light microscopy (Figs. 5.1 and 5.2), though electron microscopy usually

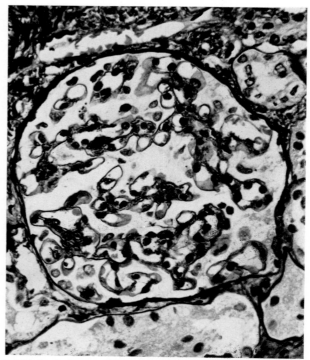

Fig. 5.2. Minimal change. The glomerulus has a fine uniform basement membrane outlining the peripheral capillary loops. P.A.S.M. × 480

reveals swelling of the epithelial cells of the glomeruli with loss of foot processes. This lesion is found in 85 per cent of children with the nephrotic syndrome in England (Cameron 1970b). Membranous lesions are characterised by a diffuse linear thickening of the glomerular capillary walls without any increase in the cellular elements of the tuft: All the glomeruli are involved and the thick capillary walls are due to dense deposits which are laid down on the epithelial aspect of the true basement membrane. This results in the production of radial projections from the basement membrane which envelop the deposits to form the thick capillary wall. The spiky basement membrane projections can be seen in sections stained with periodic acid–silver methenamine.

The third type of glomerular lesion is known as proliferative and its heterogenicity is reflected by the variety of subgroups used by different authors. The strict criterion for inclusion in this group is an increase in the cellular elements usually judged by the number of nuclei in the glomerular tufts. Estimation of proliferation is often difficult to assess because of variation in section thickness, variable degrees of glomerular involvement in one biopsy and sometimes segmental involvement. Moreover, once sclerosis has begun the proliferative element may not be evident. The increase in the number of cells may involve mesangial cells, endothelial cells or epithelial cells. In descriptive histological terms proliferative changes may be generalised, involving all or nearly all glomeruli. In such cases the lesions are usually diffuse (Figs. 5.3 and 5.4), involving the whole

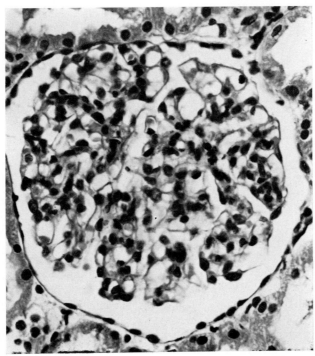

Fig. 5.3. Diffuse glomerular changes in the glomerular tuft. The increase in nuclei is mainly endothelial and mesangial. H and E. × 480

glomerular tuft, though segmental lesions involving only part of the tuft, may also be present. Cases with generalised diffuse glomerulonephritis may be classified into four subgroups (White, 1970 and Cameron, 1970*b*): acute exudative (the lesion of acute glomerulonephritis), proliferative with crescents, mesangial proliferative and membranoproliferative glomerulonephritis. Lesions of the mesangial proliferative type may be associated with an increase in mesangial matrix (Fig. 5.5) but have normal peripheral capillary loops. Such lesions are often seen in resolving post-streptococcal glomerulonephritis but may also be found in idiopathic cases of the

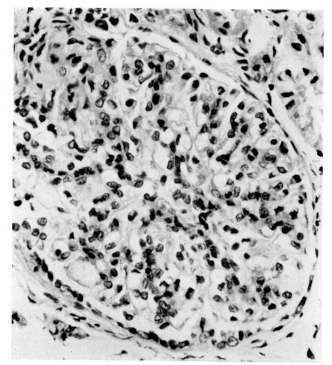

Fig. 5.4. Marked proliferative changes in the glomerular tufts
H and E. × 480

nephrotic syndrome. Membranoproliferative glomerulonephritis, sometimes called mixed membranous and proliferative, is characterised by a
proliferation of the mesangial cells and endothelial cells with a great
increase in matrix which extends around the peripheral capillary loops
producing a thick capillary wall (Figs. 5.6 and 5.7). In some cases the
glomerulus takes on a lobular appearance with a segmental nodule of
mesangial matrix forming the centre of the lobule (Fig. 5.8). These lesions
have been associated with a syndrome of hypocomplementaemia and
glomerulonephritis occurring in older children and young adults (West
et al., 1965 and Ogg et al., 1968). The lesion may, however, be seen in some
cases of post-streptococcal origin and in idiopathic forms of the nephrotic
syndrome (Burckholder et al., 1970).

   Although most cases fit into one of these categories some show intermediate features.

   The last subgroup of the proliferative lesions is also the most controversial. Focal glomerulonephritis, used in the pathological sense, indicates
a variable degree of glomerular involvement with some or many glomeruli
appearing normal. The lesions that are present may be diffuse in each tuft
but are often segmental (Figs. 5.9 and 5.10). The type of change may be
proliferative or sclerotic, though the latter may result from a proliferative

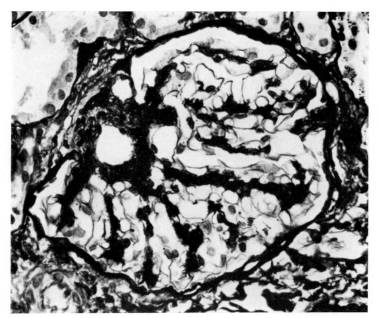

Fig. 5.5. Diffuse proliferative changes with mesangial sclerosis exaggerating the lobular stalks. The peripheral capillary basement membrane is normal. P.A.S.M. × 480

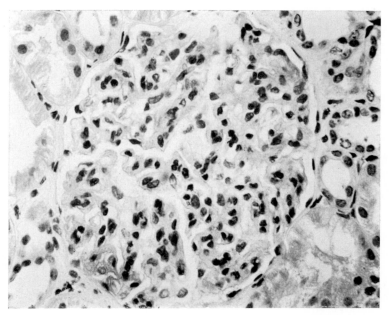

Fig. 5.6. Diffuse proliferative change in the glomerular tuft with thickening of the peripheral capillary loops. Membranoproliferative lesion. H and E. × 480

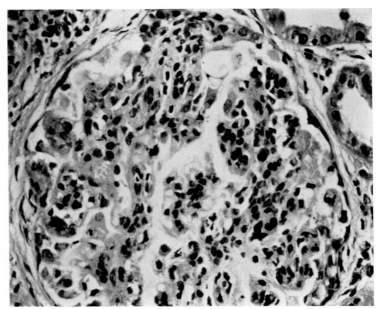

Fig. 5.7. Marked diffuse proliferative changes in the glomerular tuft with a lobular pattern and thickening of the peripheral capillary loops. H and E. × 480

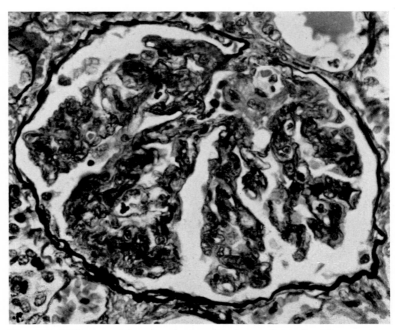

Fig. 5.8. Diffuse proliferative changes in glomerular tuft with accentuation of lobular pattern and thickening of peripheral capillary loops. P.A.S. × 480

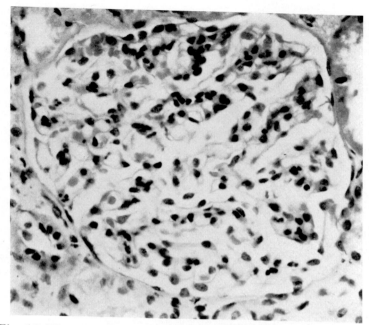

Fig. 5.9. There is a localised increase in the tuft nuclei in two segments; the nuclei are probably of mesangial and endothelial origin. H and E. × 480

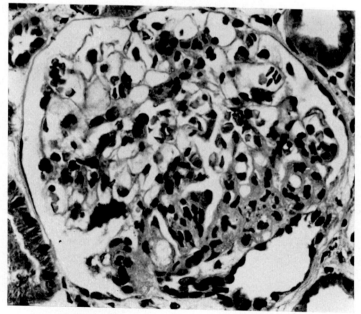

Fig. 5.10. Segmental proliferation in the glomerular tuft with local sclerosis. H and E. × 480

lesion (Figs. 5.10 and 5.11). Some authors distinguish a focal sclerotic group (White, 1970). Careful examination often reveals the lesions to be more widespread than is evident on first examination.

In some cases with focal and segmental lesions of the glomeruli there is a progressive involvement and ultimately all are abnormal.

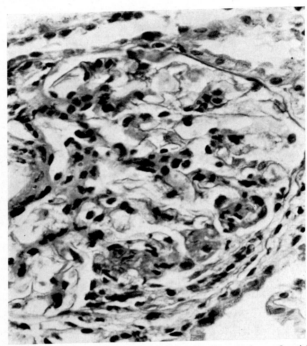

Fig. 5.11. Localised foci of sclerosis in glomerular tuft with minimal increase in nuclei. P.A.S. × 480

Histopathological features in the nephrotic syndrome due to *Plasmodium malariae*

The evidence already presented suggests that this is caused by the deposition of immune complexes in the glomeruli. The lesions produced by these complexes are those of a glomerulonephritis. The parasite itself does not play a direct role in the production of the lesion and other evidence of malaria, such as the presence of pigment in the glomeruli, is not seen. The descriptions of renal lesions in the nephrotic syndrome due to *P. malariae* are based on examination of biopsies and post mortem material from cases in which the clinical, parasitological, biochemical and immunological evidence suggests a malarial aetiology and in which there is no evidence suggesting another aetiology such as the streptococcus.

The first descriptions of these lesions in renal biopsies from children with the nephrotic syndrome in Nigeria was reported by Gilles and

Hendrickse (1963, 2 references). The pathological features of these cases were reported in detail by Edington and Mainwaring (1966) in a review of Nephropathies in West Africa. True minimal lesion was only found in 2 out of 91 biopsies examined. The majority of cases with *P. malariae* in the blood showed one of two patterns or a mixture of both. In slightly over 50 per cent there was a variable involvement of the glomeruli, often with segmental lesions. These consisted of endothelial cell glomerulitis with mesangial involvement, an increase in intercapillary P.A.S. material and occasional tuft adhesions. In the remainder the lesions were usually segmental and hyalinising with obliteration of peripheral capillary loops. The authors stressed that differentiation from post-streptococcal nephritis was often difficult (Edington and Mainwaring 1966).

In 1967 Kibukamusoke and Hutt reported their findings in cases with the nephrotic syndrome seen in Uganda in children and in adults. True minimal lesions were only seen in 3 cases and these were not associated with quartan malaria. The histological findings in Ugandan children are shown in Table 5.1. The biopsies were obtained from 53 children with an

Table 5.1

Histological findings in children with the nephrotic syndrome in Uganda

Minimal (nil) lesion	3
Proliferative lesion	
Mild generalised or focal lesions	39
Moderate or marked generalised diffuse	
proliferative lesions	11
Total	53

average age of 8 years. The quartan malarial parasite rate in this group was 71 per cent and the overall malarial parasite rate 81 per cent. Thirty-nine children had mild proliferative or focal lesions (Figs. 5.3, 5.9 and 5.10) with a variable degree of glomerular involvement, often with segmental lesions and occasionally with tuft adhesions. While the segmental lesions were sometimes proliferative, sclerotic and hyalinising lesions with mesangial and basement membrane involvement were also common (Figs. 5.11 and 5.12). Eleven cases had marked generalised diffuse lesions of the mesangial or membranoproliferative type (Figs. 5.4 and 5.6). These latter cases often showed microscopic haematuria and some degree of hypertension. In a recent review of 63 Nigerian children with the nephrotic syndrome, Hendrickse *et al.* (1972) classify 51 cases as Quartan Malarial Nephropathy. These cases were characterised by a variable number and degree of glomerular involvement and the lesions consisted of capillary wall thickening with segmental sclerosis. In those with more severe involvement, the majority of glomeruli were involved and the lesions were diffuse leading to glomerular sclerosis; this was very common in older children. The appearances appear to be similar to many of the cases described in the Uganda series as focal (Fig. 5.12).

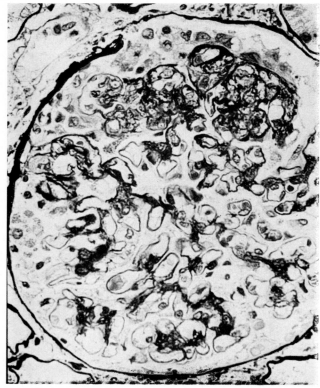

Fig. 5.12. Marked segmental lesions in two lobules with a slight increase
in mesangial matrix in some others. P.A.S.M. × 480

The histological findings in adults with the nephrotic syndrome in
Uganda were reported by Kibukamusoke and Hutt 1967. A recent review
is shown in Table 5.2.

Table 5.2

*Histological findings in adults with the nephrotic
syndrome in Uganda*

Primary glomerulonephritis	
Minimal (nil) lesion	0
Membranous lesion	10
Proliferative lesion	
Mild generalised or focal lesions	42
Moderate or marked generalised mesangial or	
membranoproliferative lesions	100
Total	152
Secondary glomerular disease	
Amyloidosis	6
Renal vein thrombosis	3
Henoch–Schonlein purpura	1
Diabetes	1
Total	11

In none of the cases with a pure membranous lesion was there any evidence to suggest a malarial aetiology; most of these patients were in the older age groups. True minimal lesion was not seen in adults, though some of the focal cases had to be searched carefully to reveal the lesion. Although the parasite levels were not as high in these adult cases, *P. malariae* was found more frequently than in controls and other immunological evidence pointed to this aetiology in most cases.

Twelve cases with generalised and diffuse lesions had clinicopathological evidence of streptococcal infection, four of these had marked crescent formation, a feature never seen in cases thought to be of malarial origin (Wing, Kibukamusoke and Hutt, 1971). Immunological evidence suggesting malarial aetiology was found in some cases with membranoproliferative lesions.

It is apparent that adults who develop the nephrotic syndrome in Uganda are more likely to have marked glomerular lesions than children and that many, if not the majority, of these cases also have a malarial aetiology. The higher frequency of proliferative lesion in adults is also evident from the U.K. and elsewhere (Cameron, 1970a). The factors that determine the glomerular response to injury are still unknown and age may affect the aetiological agents and, or the host response.

Progression of the disease and relationship of the nephrotic syndrome due to *P. malariae* to chronic glomerulonephritis

Autopsy studies in Uganda have shown that chronic glomerulonephritis is a common cause of death and that the majority of patients with severe hypertension under 40 years of age who die in hospital have this condition (Hutt and Coles, 1969). Some of these cases are undoubtedly post-streptococcal in origin and outbreaks of acute exudative glomerulonephritis have been recorded in Uganda (Hutt and White, 1964). It is thought that the majority, however, are the late results of glomerulonephritis due to *Plasmodium malariae* and a number of cases have been followed through the nephrotic stage to the stage of chronic renal failure and death; most of these cases have been in their second or third decade. Longitudinal studies in a group of cases where renal biopsies were repeated after intervals have shown that cases with mild and focal lesions may become protein-free with treatment; some, however, persist with proteinuria for several years with very little deterioration or alteration in the renial biopsy appearances (Wing, Hutt and Kibukamusoke, 1972). Cases with generalised diffuse glomerulonephritis may also remain unchanged over several years and run a fluctuating course: those with membranoproliferative lesions are more likely to progress to chronic renal failure. Long-term studies on many cases are still required to work out the natural history of the disease in relation to age, type and progression of glomerular lesion and response to therapy.

Electron microscopy

As might be expected from the variable appearance on light microscopy, there are considerable variations in the glomerular appearances on electron microscopy. Allison *et al.* (1969) describe moderate thickening of the basement membrane and circumscribed dense deposits beneath the epithelium (Figs. 5.13 and 5.14). In such cases the foot processes were usually

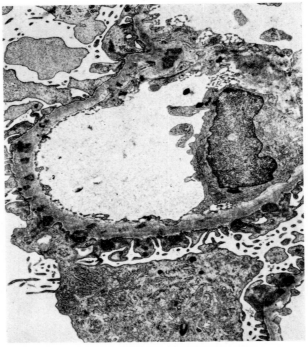

Fig. 5.13. Electron micrograph showing finger-like projections of endothelial cells and deposits in the basement membrane beneath the epithelium. × 10,000. (From Allison A. C., 1969. *Lancet*, **i**, 1232.)

free but were occasionally fused and there was a zone of increased electron density in the epithelial foot processes immediately adjacent to the basement membrane. In other cases they report an irregular thickening of the basement membrane with variable areas of increased and decreased electron density. Most of these cases showed fusion of the foot processes of the epithelial cells and both epithelial and endothelial cells were frequently increased in numbers. Hendrickse *et al.* 1972 describe the electron microscopy in 22 patients from West Africa. Discrete subepithelial deposits were not identified in this group and the essential abnormality consisted of an increased amount of basement membrane-like material, arranged in a plexiform manner in the subendothelial region. They also noted small lacunae scattered through the basement membrane, which they considered to be a unique feature.

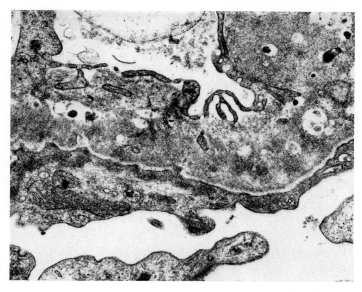

Fig. 5.14. Electron micrograph showing pronounced thickening of the basement membrane, fusion of foot processes and an area of increased electron density alongside the basement membrane. × 24,000. (From Allison A. C., 1969. *Lancet* **i**, 1232.)

BIBLIOGRAPHY

Allison, A. C., Houba, V., Hendrickse, R. G., Edington, G. M., de Petris, S. and Adeniyi, A. (1969). Immune complexes in the nephrotic syndrome of African children. *Lancet*, i, 1232.

Burkholder, P. M., Marchand, A. and Krueger, R. P. (1970). Mixed membranous and proliferative glomerulonephritis. *Lab. Invest.*, **23**, 459.

Cameron, J. S. (1970a). Nephrotic syndrome. *Brit. med. J.*, **4**, 350.

— (1970b). Glomerulonephritis. *Brit. med. J.*, **4**, 285.

Edington, G. M. and Mainwaring, A. R. (1966). Nephropathies in West Africa. *International Academy of Pathology Monograph No. 6.* Williams and Wilkins, Baltimore.

Gilles, H. M. and Hendrickse, R. G. (1963). Nephrosis in Nigerian children. *Brit. med. J.*, **2**, 27.

Hendrickse, R. G. and Gilles, H. M. (1963). The nephrotic syndrome and other renal diseases in children in Western Nigeria. *E. Afr. med. J.*, **40**, 186.

Hendrickse, R. G., White, R. H. R., Edington, G. M., Houba, V., Glasgow, E. F. and Adeniyi, A. (1972). Quartan malarial nephrotic syndrome. *Lancet* i, 1163.

Hutt, M. S. R. and Coles, R. (1969). Postmortem findings in hypertensive subjects in Kampala, Uganda. *E. Afr. med. J.*, **46**, 342.

Hutt, M. S. R. and White, R. H. R. (1964). A clinico-pathological study of acute glomerulonephritis in East African children. *Arch. Dis. Childh.*, **39**, 313.

Kibukamusoke, J. W. and Hutt, M. S. R. (1967). Histological features of the nephrotic syndrome associated with quartan malaria. *J. clin. Path.*, **20**, 117.

Ogg, C. S., Cameron, J. S. and White, R. H. R. (1968). The C′3 component of complement (β_{1C}-globulin) in patients with heavy proteinuria. *Lancet*, ii, 78.

West, C. D., McAdams, A. J., McConville, J. M., Davies, N. C. and Holland, N. H. (1965). Hypocomplementemic and normocomplementemic persistent (chronic) glomerulonephritis. *J. Pediat.*, **67,** 1089.

White, R. H. R. (1970). Glomerulonephritis in children. *Brit. J. Hosp. Med.*, **3,** 746.

Wing, A. J., Kibukamusoke, J. W. and Hutt, M. S. R. (1971). Poststreptococcal glomerulonephritis and the nephrotic syndrome in Uganda. *Trans. roy. Soc. trop. Med. Hyg.*, **65,** 543.

Wing, A. J., Hutt, M. S. R. and Kibukamusoke, J. W. (1972). Progression and remission in the nephrotic syndrome associated with quartan malaria in Uganda. *Quart. J. Med.* **41,** 273.

6 Immunology

In Chapter 4 evidence was given for an association between *Plasmodium malariae* and the nephrotic syndrome. This association was shown to be a direct one, namely *P. malariae* playing a causative part in the production of the nephrotic syndrome. The features of this syndrome were shown to be so peculiar in several respects that Kibukamusoke, Hutt and Wilks (1967) recommended the use of the term 'Nephrotic Syndrome of Quartan Malaria' when referring to this disease entity.

Evidence has accumulated in the last few years to confirm the concept of this disease as an entity. The association with *P. malariae* in a direct way and the absence of malaria parasites in biopsies or other material from the kidney of affected patients led to suggestions that renal damage might be due to immune processes (Gilles and Hendrickse, 1963; Kibukamusoke, 1966a, b). The mechanism by which damage occurs in the kidney has excited a great deal of interest and valuable work has consequently been done.

Elevation of malaria antibodies in the serum

In a study of malaria antibody titres in patients with this syndrome, Kibukamusoke and others (1967) found a significant increase in titres among patients when compared with sera from matched controls (Fig. 6.1). This situation occurred despite considerable losses of identifiable malaria antibodies in the urine of nephrotic patients (Kibukamusoke and Wilks, 1965a, b). The severity of urinary loss correlated well with the concentration of malaria antibodies in the serum. This loss causes a considerable decapitation of antibody titres at peak values. Without this loss the difference between antibody concentrations in nephrotics would be even more significantly different from controls.

The presence of malaria parasites in a context of increased serum antibodies suggested that the antigen-excess situation of Dixon (Dixon *et al.*, 1958; Dixon, 1962–63, 1968) might be the operative mechanism (Kibukamusoke, 1966a, 1969). Dixon's theory postulates that, in immunological states where there is a slight excess of antigen over antibody, antigen–antibody complexes may be found in active circulation and that these (soluble) complexes may be deposited in the kidney and cause immunological damage (Unanue and Dixon, 1967b).

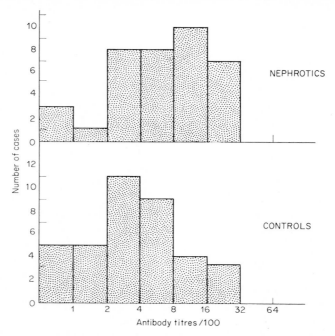

Fig. 6.1. Malaria antibodies among nephrotics and matched controls.
The proportion of cases with a titre in excess of 1:800 in the two groups
is significantly different at the 5 per cent level (χ^2 test)

Evidence for immune complexes in the circulation

It now remained for these complexes to be demonstrated in the serum of sufferers. Some evidence for this was reported soon afterwards by Soothill and Hendrickse (1967) when they detected the presence of a complement component, βIC, in the first peak of 'Sephadex G-200' gel filtration of the serum of some of the children suffering from the disease in Nigeria. This finding suggested that complement 'was incorporated into a macromolecular form as would be anticipated if it were bound to soluble antigen–antibody complexes'. These workers also found that the complement component was present in the altered form in many of the cases suggesting that it had been involved in an immunological reaction (Soothill, 1967; Linscott and Cochrane, 1964).

Studies of relevant sera by Professor J. Hardwicke in Birmingham, England, were unable to confirm these findings. Employing sera from 14 Ugandan cases using column chromatographic analysis none showed evidence of IgG in the first peak of elution (Fig. 6.2). All the first peaks were then concentrated and run on Sephadex G-200 (Fig. 6.2 last box) and here again all IgG was in its usual position. It was therefore concluded that no significant IgG complexes were circulating in the sera of these

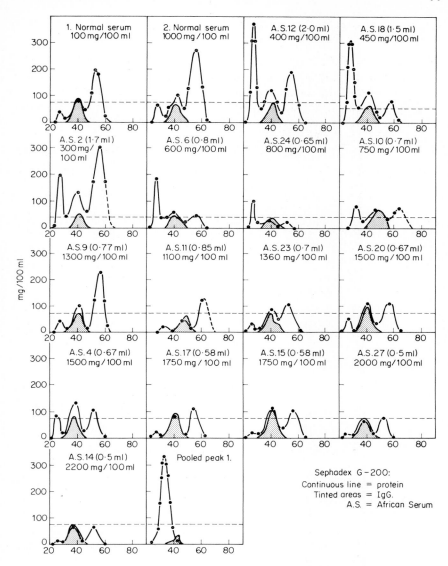

Fig. 6.2. Sephadex chromatographic analysis of sera from 14 patients with nephrotic syndrome of quartan malaria and 2 controls

patients. This, however, did not exclude the possibility of IgM complexes being present. Further work is now being planned for a search of IgM complexes possibly by ultracentrifugal separation and subsequent detection by fluorescent techniques.

Deposition of immune complexes on the glomerular basement membrane

The deposition of these soluble complexes in the glomeruli was first demonstrated by Ward and Kibukamusoke (1969) in a study of frozen kidney tissue obtained from patients suffering from this syndrome at Mulago Hospital, Kampala, Uganda. These workers, using fluorescent antibody staining techniques on frozen renal tissues, found glomerular deposits of human IgM, IgG, IgA as well as complement component (βIC) and fibrin in many cases; IgM predominated and complement was always found in association with immunoglobulins. A total of 30 cases were studied and the results are given in Table 6.1.

Table 6.1

Immunoglobulin studies in renal biopsies from patients with the nephrotic syndrome of quartan malaria

	Number of cases	Number positive	Positive (%)	Comment
Total	30	26	87	
IgM		18	60	Predominant with heaviest deposits
IgG		11	37	Usually faint deposits
IgA		3	10	Faint deposits
βIC		11	37	Always in combination with immunoglobulin
Fibrin		4	13	Its presence unimpressive

The pattern of immune complex deposition was consistently irregular nodular and beaded (Figs. 6.3 and 6.4) though Houba *et al.* (1970) also describe a 'mixed' type. The deposits accurately outlined the basement membrane of the glomeruli. This pattern is characteristic of deposition of pre-formed antigen–antibody complexes on the glomerular basement membrane (Dixon, 1962–3; 1968; Weigle, 1964; Unanue and Dixon, 1967*b*). Fluorescence was mainly found in the glomeruli (Ward and Kibukamusoke, 1969; Adeniyi *et al.*, 1970).

Figures 6.5–6.8 show the same glomerulus stained for IgG, IgM, βIC and *P. malariae* antigen. It is apparent that the territorial distribution of these deposits is similar.

The linear pattern associated with glomerular basement membrane antigenicity was not seen in any of these cases, though it was found in kidneys which were the seat of glomerulonephritis due to other causes which we studied at the same time. Adeniyi *et al.* (1970) while confirming these findings reported that some of their cases, studied in a similar manner,

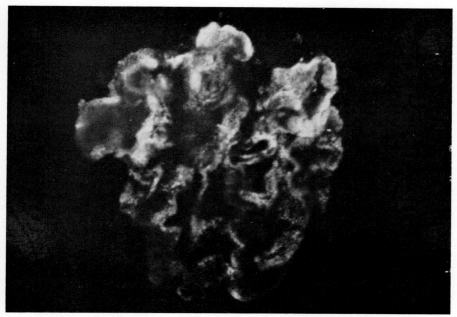

Fig. 6.3. Irregular, granular and beaded deposits outlining the glomerular basement membrane. × 600.

changed to the linear pattern of fluorescence during the course of immuno-suppressive therapy. This point will be discussed later in this chapter. The territorial distribution of immunoglobulins, complement and antigen was similar (Figs. 6.5–6.8), suggesting pre-formation before deposition.

Patterns of Fluorescence

The classical coarse granular pattern of fluorescence is present in the majority of patients but a finer diffuse pattern is also seen. Houba (1971) found it in about 20 per cent of patients and there were no differences due to age or sex.

The diffuse pattern was however seen much more frequently among adults with long standing disease and also tended to occur among those with severer disease at all ages. The pattern was associated with a significantly lower incidence of complement binding and IgM ($P < 0.01$), though IgG was as frequently seen among those with this pattern as among those with the diffuse and 'mixed' types.

Six out of 11 patients in Houba's series (Houba, 1971) who showed the diffuse pattern had IgG_2 deposits. Conversely all patients with the granular pattern showed IgG_3 except one. Only one showing a diffuse pattern had this immunoglobulin subclass.

The prevalence of IgG and IgM was similar in the granular and 'mixed' patterns of fluorescence and most of the patients with the granular pattern were complement positive. Findings in the tubules were not so clear cut.

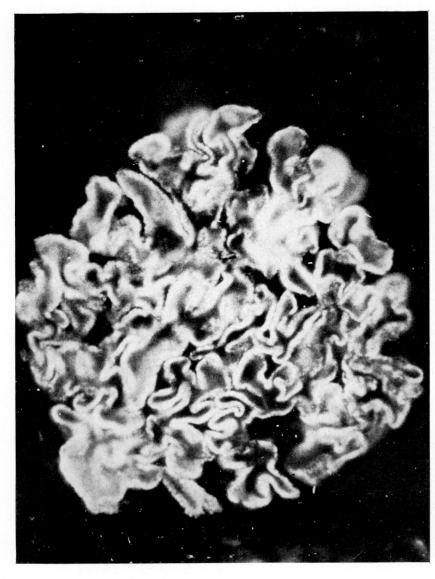

Fig. 6.4. Heavy IgG deposits along glomerular basement membranes in a beaded, nodular pattern. × 400. (Ward, P. A. and Kibukamusoke, J. W., 1969. *Lancet*, **i**, 283.)

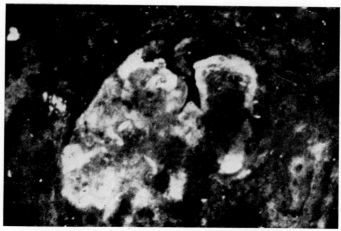

Fig. 6.5. Renal biopsy from another nephrotic child with quartan malaria. Heavy γG deposits are irregularly scattered in glomerulus. × 600. (From Ward, P. A. and Conran, P. B. 1969. *Milit. Med.* **134**, 10, 1228)

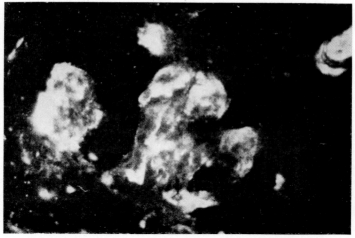

Fig. 6.6. Serial section of that in Fig. 6.5 stained for human γM. × 600. (From Ward, P. A. and Conran, P. B. 1969. *Milit. Med.* **134**, 10, 1228)

Houba (1971) found that fluorescence due to complement was always granular but less widely distributed than immunoglobulin fluorescence in the same glomerulus. Sometimes it was focal or limited to parts of the glomerulus. A higher incidence of complement deposition was found in males.

Tubular Fluorescence

Houba, Allison and others (1970) studying immunofluorescence in the nephrotic syndrome of quartan malaria found positive granular staining with anti-globulin and/for anti-complement conjugates in the tubules in a third of their patients. The deposits were found between the lumen and

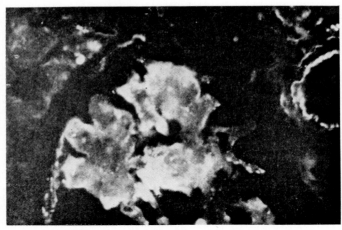

Fig. 6.7. Serial section of that in Fig. 6.5 stained for human C3. Auto-fluorescence is seen in internal elastic lamina of artery (upper right). × 600. (From Ward, P. A. and Conran, P. B. (1969). *Milit. Med.* **134**, 10, 1228)

the nuclei of tubular cells. In a later study Houba (1971) found tubular fluorescence in an increased percentage (56 per cent) in adult patients. The figure remained 30 per cent in childhood cases. The immunoglobulin in this situation was almost invariably IgG though IgM was demonstrated in a few cases. Granular patterns were associated with pure IgG fluorescence while diffuse patterns tended to appear when IgG and IgM were both present.

In a further study (Houba *et al.*, 1971) IgG and IgM were found in tubules of 17 of the 50 patients they studied. In 5 of these patients complement was additionally present while *P. malariae* antigen was found in 11 of 36 cases. This was in contrast to 9 out of 36 patients examined for glomerular *P. malariae* antigen.

A higher incidence of tubular fluorescence was found in repeat biopsies from patients who had failed to respond to antimalarials (given singly), steroids or cyclophosphamide although there was no significant change in glomerular fluorescence (Houba *et al.*, 1971).

The antigen

The demonstration of antigen–antibody complexes begs the question of which antigen? Unanue and Dixon (1967b) reported that glomerulonephritis due to deposition of soluble complexes occurred with deposits bearing an antigen which was immunologically dissimilar to basement membrane protein. The occurrence of these deposits in the nephropathy associated with quartan malaria was therefore not surprising. It suggested that the antigen is derived from or produced by the malaria parasite.

In Chapter 4 evidence was presented to show that *P. malariae* was the only parasite associated with the causation of malarial nephrotic syndrome. This suggested that this parasite harboured or produced a peculiar protein which other human plasmodia neither had nor produced. Allison *et al.* (1969) confirm this. Ward and Kibukamusoke (1969) searched for such an antigen from frozen renal biopsies obtained from active cases. These cases were shown to have deposits of immune complexes at the time by immunofluorescent staining techniques. It was impossible, however, to demonstrate the presence of any malarial antigen using polyvalent sera though these sera bore high titres of malaria antibodies. The sera were obtained from immune malarial subjects at Mulago, Kampala, Uganda. Some of them were obtained from active cases of the nephrotic syndrome who had shown numerous parasites of *P. malariae* in blood slides. The search was equally unsuccessful even after attempts at 'unmasking' the antigen using differential elution techniques with potassium thiocyanate or acid (citrate) buffers (Edgington *et al.*, 1968). The rationale of this work was the possibility that reaction sites might be covered up by the large amounts of antibody in the deposits (Dixon *et al.*, 1967). However, the use of an apparently monovalent serum for *P. malariae* obtained from a patient infected with this parasite after a fresh outbreak of pure *P. malariae* malaria following a long period of freedom from malaria in Ceylon yielded positive results from three cases.* Houba and others (1970) were also able to demonstrate positive staining with anti-*P. malariae* conjugate in a third of their cases.

Table 6.2

Detection of P. malariae *antigen immunofluorescence*

Indicator agent*	Result
1. Labelled high antibody serum to *P. malariae*	Positive
2. Labelled serum with no antibody to *P. malariae*	Negative
3. Labelled high antibody serum to Rubeola Virus	Negative
4. Labelled high antibody serum to *P. cynomolgi*	Negative

* All are human sera except for one that bears the simian antibody to *P. cynomolgi*.

Ward and Conran (1969) in further work on the subject of identification of the antigen presumed to reside in the complexes deposited in the glomeruli studied 31 splenectomised monkeys on whom they had performed a unilateral nephrectomy and infected with *P. cynomolgi*. Nephropathy is not normally a symptom of *P. cynomolgi* infections and the rationale of unilateral nephrectomy was 'in order to increase the amount of circulating immune complexes perfusing the remaining kidney'. Splenectomy was performed in order to permit an increase in parasite density. The result was that approximately two-thirds of the animals developed renal deposits instead of the usual 15 per cent in non-surgically prepared animals.

* This serum from Ceylon was highly specific for *P. malariae* (Table 6.2).

In this study Ward and Conran found that glomerular immune deposition occurred during the two periods of peak parasitaemia. The first occurred between the 7th and 11th day after infection at a time when 'antigen or parasite elimination' occurred. Twenty-five to 100 per cent of renal biopsies were positive for complexes at this time (Fig. 6.9). These

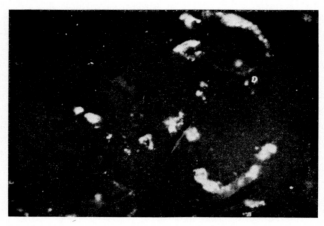

Fig. 6.8. Serial section of that in Fig. 6.5 stained for antigen of *P. malariae*. The distribution is granular, less intense but similar to pattern of γG, γM and C3. × 600. (From Ward, P. A. and Conran, P. B. 1969. *Milit. Med.* **134,** 10, 1228)

deposits persisted for a brief period of 2 or 3 days only. The second period of deposition again coincided with the second peak of parasitaemia (Fig. 6.9) from day 15 through the next 2 weeks—a sustained secondary peak. Deposits were invariable during days 20 to 22 and absent when the parasite density was lowest between the primary and secondary peaks.

The deposits in the glomeruli consisted of monkey IgG and C'3 along glomerular capillary walls in an irregular granular pattern and involving most of the glomeruli. No deposits were seen in tubules or in other extraglomerular areas.

The search for malarial antigen revealed scattered intact parasites in renal glomerular capillaries as well as in the pericapillary tubules (Ward and Conran, 1969). There was only slight evidence of a granular deposition of malarial antigen in a pattern similar to that of IgG and C'3, but, when found, the deposits of malarial antigen were always in association with those of IgG and C'3. This finding gives very strong support to the contention that the deposits are preformed and then laid down as 'antigen–antibody–complement macromolecules'. The demonstration of intact parasites in glomeruli has not so far been made in man and this has led to the suggestion that it is an antigen from the parasite that is involved rather than the parasite itself.

The occurrence of deposits only during periods of dense parasitaemia

is of interest as increased parasite density would facilitate their demonstration. In the human subject, however, this may not always be true as several
attempts have had to be made employing special techniques for the

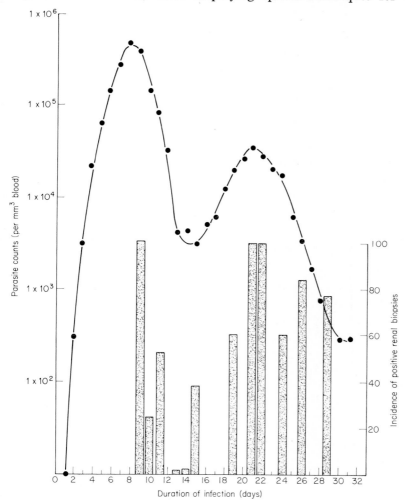

Fig. 6.9. Parasitaemia levels of *P. cynomolgi* in monkeys infected on day
0. Vertical bars represent incidence of immunofluorescent deposits in
renal glomeruli. (From Ward P. A. and Conran P. B. 1969. *Milit. Med.*
134, 10, 1228)

demonstration of parasites particularly in the adult patient (Kibukamusoke,
1967). This observation may help to explain the apparent intermittent
appearance of parasitaemia (Kibukamusoke, 1967). It has further been
observed in several cases who have been followed up for up to 8 years in
the Renal Clinic at Mulago Hospital, Kampala, Uganda, that recurrences
may be due to reappearance of parasites in the blood—either by reinfection
or by relapse (Fig. 7.1, p. 103).

McGregor *et al.* (1968) reported the presence of soluble antigens in the serum of children and an adult woman (recently delivered of a child) suffering or convalescing from acute and heavy infections of *P. falciparum.* Their investigations showed that these antigens were not all identical though they were probably malarial (*P. falciparum*) in origin. In none of the cases was it possible to detect the antigen for more than 28 days though it persisted for as short as 3 days after patent parasitaemia in some cases. In some of the children it appeared as though there were more than one antigen present in the serum. Extracts from placental schizonts (*P. falciparum*) were also shown to contain considerable quantities of plasmodial antigen. McGregor and his co-workers (1968), however, thought that these antigens were poorly immunogenic.

Zuckerman (1969) has been able to show that plasmodia contain several antigens each capable of giving rise to a specific antibody in an experimental animal.

In 1970 Wilson and Voller found malarial antigens in the sera of owl monkeys at the height of infection with *Plasmodium falciparum.* The antigens were identical with certain malarial S-antigens present in the sera of West African (Gambian) children acutely infected with *P. falciparum.* This work has opened a new chapter in experimental malariology by providing an experimental model which is relevant to the study of the serology of human malaria. Voller now has owl monkeys infected with *P. malariae* and it is hoped that parallel studies will be done on this problem in due course.

Antibodies to these antigens were almost universally present in adults (96·0 per cent) and the sera usually contained antibodies to several of these soluble antigens (McGregor *et al.*, 1968). Only 20·5 per cent of the children showed presence of these antibodies. In each instance the reaction developed between the plasma sample of an aparasitaemic adult and that of a young child intensely infected with *P. falciparum.*

Studies of the physicochemical nature of the soluble antigens suggest that they are proteins of high molecular weight (about 300,000–900,000) (Turner, 1967). However, fractionation of 'immune' sera on Sephadex G-200 indicated that the gel-precipitin antibodies to the soluble antigens belong to the IgG class (McGregor *et al.*, 1968).

Eaton (1939) also found a soluble antigen in the serum of monkeys heavily parasitised with *P. Knowlesi* and when the antigen was injected into normal monkeys it stimulated the production of antibodies 'similar to those produced as a sequel to malarial infection, but conferred no protection against plasmodial challenge'. More recently an antigen was also found in the serum of monkeys heavily parasitised with *P. Knowlesi.* This antigen reacted with sera from animals convalescent from malarial infection in gel-precipitation tests (Cox, 1966).

It is interesting that the only adult case in which this type of soluble antigen was found was in a state of pregnancy—a state in which women are more susceptible to malaria (Gilles *et al.*, 1969). The immunological status in the state of pregnancy with reference to malaria may thus be similar to that present during childhood. It may not be surprising therefore that pregnancy should worsen malarial nephropathy (Kibukamusoke, Hutt and Wilks, 1967).

The finding of a soluble antigen in a child suffering from a severe infection of *P. malariae* is thus very interesting (Allison *et al.*, 1969). A similar antigen was found in eluates from the kidney of a child who succumbed from quartan malarial nephrosis (Allison *et al.*, 1969). This antigen was not present in the spleen of a child who died of a heavy *P. falciparum* infection. It is therefore possible that this is truly the antigen that has eluded workers in this field before.

Persistence of antigen–antibody complexes in the circulation

It has been amply demonstrated in experimental work that chronic glomerulonephritis can be produced by continued injection of sera containing antigen–antibody complexes (Unanue and Dixon, 1967a, b). The same is true of rabbits receiving daily injections of a heterologous protein for prolonged periods of time (Weigle, 1964). These rabbits produced barely enough antibody to combine with all antigen and therefore contained high levels of circulating antigen–antibody complexes. These animals developed a chronic progressive glomerulonephritis either proliferative or membranous, associated with oedema, uraemia, proteinuria and hypercholesterolaemia (Weigle, 1964). Conditions favouring persistence of these complexes would therefore be expected to lead to chronic glomerulonephritis.

There is considerable evidence that the average size of soluble immune complexes plays a crucial role in determining the persistence of the complexes within the circulation (Heidelberger and Pedersen, 1937; Pappenheimer *et al.*, 1940; Eisen and Karush, 1949; Morrack *et al.*, 1951; Singer and Campbell, 1951, 1952, 1955; Oncley *et al.*, 1952; Becker, 1953; Karush, 1956; Weigle and Maurer, 1957; Weigle, 1964). When antigen–antibody precipitates formed at equivalence were injected into rabbits, both the antigen and antibody components were rapidly eliminated from the blood but, conversely, certain soluble antigen–antibody complexes prepared with excess antigen persisted in the circulation in a manner similar to the complexes formed early during a primary antibody response (Weigle, 1958; Weigle, 1964). The smaller complexes which predominate in the region of extreme antigen excess remained in the circulation longest (Weigle, 1964), and it was of no material consequence whether the antibody used was of a precipitating or non-precipitating type (Weigle, 1964).

The progression of the glomerular lesion in quartan malarial nephropathy (Kibukamusoke, 1968) is reminiscent of the situation just described. Chronic cases have been reported to show the classical pattern of soluble complex deposition in the glomeruli on immunofluorescence staining, particularly if they showed overt signs of activity (Ward and Kibukamusoke, 1969). It is therefore very likely that one of the mechanisms leading to progression is the persistence of circulating soluble immune complexes.

The persistence of parasitaemia in chronic malaria has been shown to be largely due to parasite variation (Brown and Brown, 1965; Voller and Rossan, 1969; Cox, 1959; Wellde and Sadun, 1967; Weigle, 1964). This persistence of parasitaemia may create the conditions necessary for prolonged interaction between 'antigen' and antibody with the formation of soluble immune complexes over a prolonged period of time. As the balance between antigen and antibody is vital for the formation of persisting complexes urinary loss of antibody (Kibukamusoke and Wilks, 1965a, b) may be an important event in this connection. In their studies, these workers found that the severity of loss was a function of the serum antibody titre. The loss is therefore heavier the higher the serum titre is. This loss may operate like an equilibration mechanism for the maintenance of a given titre in the serum thus enhancing the formation of complexes of the correct size.

Dixon and others (1961) and Andres and his co-workers (1963) reported that two-thirds of their rabbits receiving daily injections of antigen and making a large antibody response developed an acute proliferative glomerulonephritis which was similar in all respects to that of 'one-shot' serum sickness. The nephritis developed at a time when the rabbits were beginning to make antibody and thus passing from an antigen excess to an antibody excess situation. In these circumstances they were exposed to circulating complexes. When a state of antibody excess had been established, the nephritis subsided. This observation may account for the response of Boyd's cases (1940) to antimalarials. Such a happy result, however, has only been reported in non-immune patients to malaria. The response to antimalarials is singularly absent in humans with previous malaria experience (Gilles and Hendrickse, 1963; Kibukamusoke, Hutt and Wilks, 1967). However, it may also be the explanation for the short-lived proteinuria of malaria fever.

Almost all the rabbits which had mild to moderate antibody responses developed chronic glomerulonephritis (Dixon et al., 1961; Andres et al., 1963). Most of these rabbits were in slight antigen excess for 1–14 weeks before proteinuria developed. In many rabbits the development of nephritis could be accelerated or retarded at will by varying the dose of antigen.

Clinically the glomerulonephritis was characterised by moderate to severe proteinuria, cylindruria, hypoproteinaemia, hyperlipaemia and elevated blood urea nitrogen. By optical microscopy the kidneys showed varying degrees of endothelial cell proliferation, basement membrane thickening and polymorphonuclear accumulation. These features are the same as those observed in the human disease (Chapter 2). Unlike the human disease, however, severely nephritic rabbits showed epithelial crescents (Wing, Hutt and Kibukamusoke (1972); Kibukamusoke and Hutt, 1967). In contrast, human cases show increased antibody production (Kibukamusoke, Hutt and Wilks, 1967). The increased amount of antibody in human cases, however, may mean that they are of low affinity.

By fluorescent antibody methods the antigen, host gammaglobulin, apparently specific antibody and βIC-globulin were localised in the glomerular capillary walls as dense bead-like deposits along the basement membranes—findings also reported in the human disease (Ward and Kibukamusoke, 1969; Allison et al., 1969; Adeniyi et al., 1970). A correlation was established between the appearance and amount of these immunological deposits in the glomeruli and the appearance and degree of proteinuria and of basement membrane thickening seen by optical microscopy. These immune complexes seen by the fluorescent antibody technique appeared to correspond with dense amorphous masses of varying sizes seen by electron microscopy along the epithelial side of the basement membrane (Unanue and Dixon, 1967b), a feature also described in the human disease (Allison et al., 1969). Andres et al. (1963), using the ferritin antibody technique, demonstrated the presence of antigen in these masses ultrastructurally. This observation conformed to the finding of malaria antigen in the deposits of some of the patients with the human disease (Ward and Kibukamusoke, 1969).

Dixon and others (1961) reported that once the glomerulonephritis was fully established, cessation of antigen injections caused partial, but not complete, reversal of the clinical and pathological symptoms. In our experience at Mulago Hospital one interesting feature that we have repeatedly observed is the persistence of the syndrome after elimination of parasitaemia in patients with as short a period as 5 days. Dixon and his colleagues' observation therefore is in direct conformity with ours that once the disease becomes established removal of the antigen does not lead to remission.

The immune complexes noted in the glomeruli at the height of the disease diminished very slowly after cessation of injections but were never seen to disappear completely (Dixon et al., 1961) and their rate of removal was uninfluenced by administration of steroids (Dixon et al., 1965). Clinical observation in the human disease has revealed that a full remission is associated with disappearance of the immune complex deposits from the glomeruli whether this be spontaneous or therapeutically induced (Ward and Kibukamusoke, 1969; Adeniyi et al., 1970). The failure of steroids to remove deposits is in conformity with the clinical observation of steroid resistance. The half-disappearance time of antigen from animal kidneys was 1–2 weeks (Dixon et al., 1965), but the available evidence suggests that this is very much longer in the human subject.

Several other findings are consistent with observations in the nephrotic syndrome of quartan malaria in humans. In a follow-up study of many cases at the Renal Clinic in Mulago Hospital, I reported that a number of cases progressed and after variable periods of time died in uraemia with or without hypertension (Kibukamusoke, 1968; 1969). I also consider that this syndrome is largely responsible for the high incidence of renal hypertension in the tropics.

Chronic glomerulonephritis has also been induced in rats by chronic administration of human serum albumin (Fennell et al., 1965). The disease was similar in all respects to the disease in rabbits.

Mice of the NZB strain are prone to spontaneous development of a Coombs-positive haemolytic anaemia, hepatosplenomegaly and anti-nuclear antibodies (Helyer and Howie, 1963; Holmes and Barnett, 1963). Some of the diseased mice also developed a severe chronic glomerulo-nephritis (Helyer and Howie, 1963; Aarons, 1964; Howie and Helyer, 1965). The disease is believed to be autoimmune comparable to systemic lupus erythematosus and immunofluorescent techniques have demonstrated granular deposits of soluble complex nephritis along the glomerular basement membrane (Aarons, 1964). Electron microscopy has also revealed sub-epithelial deposits similar to serum sickness nephritis (Unanue and Dixon, 1967b).

Of interest in this connection are Greenwood, Herrick and Voller's observations (1970) and also Greenwood and Voller (1970a) when a suppression of the autoimmune disease in these mice was induced by infection with malaria. They infected a strain of B/W mice with *Plasmodium berghei yoelli* at an early stage and were able to demonstrate protection against the development of renal disease. These workers (Greenwood and Voller, 1970b) further demonstrated a delay of the onset of a positive Coombs Test in NZB mice by malaria infection. The renal disease which these mice suffer, however, appeared to have been aggravated. These observations are curious and interesting but difficult to explain at present.

Serum complement in the nephrotic syndrome of quartan malaria

There is now considerable evidence from a study of renal biopsies and of sera from patients with the nephropathy of *P. malariae* infection to suggest that soluble antigen–antibody complexes are involved in the production or maintenance of the renal lesions. This evidence has been reviewed in the preceding pages. Low serum complement and $C'3$ component concentrations have been reported in active nephritides thought to arise from soluble complex deposition in the kidney: serum sickness (Weigle and Dixon, 1958), acute post-streptococcal glomerulonephritis (West, Northway and Davis, 1964) and lupus nephritis (Christian, 1969). The measurement of complement concentrations in this disease is therefore of interest.

Cameron and Kibukamusoke (1971) measured plasma $C'3$ concentrations in 24 patients with the nephrotic syndrome of quartan malaria. These patients were in different stages of the disease: active, progressive, chronic and full remission.

Results from a radial diffusion method (Ogg, Cameron and White, 1968) indicated that the levels were unaltered and fell in the normal range. Using a non-parametric test for significance it was found that the difference between active cases of the nephrotic syndrome and controls was not statistically significant. Nor was the difference between remission, progressive and control cases. These results were somewhat surprising as Soothill and Hendrickse (1967) had found not only binding of complement in macromolecular form but also its alteration to the βIA form indicating participation in an immunological reaction. Depletion of serum haemolytic complements was shown to occur at a time of immune elimination (the period in which immune complexes form) in one-shot serum sickness (Schwab et al., 1950; Moll and Hawn, 1952; Weigle and Dixon, 1958; Rhyne and Germuth, 1961). However, certain antibody–antigen complexes which are formed in vivo during a primary antibody response to a foreign protein are incapable of reducing the level of circulating complement (Linscott and Cochrane, 1964) and this may be true of those of quartan malarial nephropathy.

Of interest is Ngu and Monekosso's work (1968) in Lagos where I had previously studied this syndrome and found the presentation to be identical with experiences at Mulago Hospital (Kibukamusoke, 1966a). These workers confirmed my findings on steroid and immuno-suppressive therapy. They found certain components of serum complement to be lowered in about 70 per cent of cases on admission. The levels returned to normal in 'practically all cases' who achieved a full remission on immuno-suppressive therapy.

Possible biphasic immunological reaction in the glomeruli

The failure of quartan malarial nephropathy to resolve on antimalarial therapy is puzzling, but may mean that the antigen responsible for the formation of immune complexes is separate from the parasite itself. The work of Allison and others (1969) suggests that this is so. However, the known soluble antigens occurring in association with P. falciparum malaria parasitaemia do not tend to persist in circulation after elimination of parasitaemia (MacGregor et al., 1968). Whether those due to P. malariae (Allison et al., 1969) persist for longer periods is unknown.

Boyd (1940), however, appears to have obtained a true response to antimalarial therapy in his non-immune cases and it is possible that 'resistance' to antimalarials is confined to immune (to malaria) subjects only.

We know that a remission of proteinuria is associated with the disappearance of immune deposits from the glomeruli (Ward and Kibukamusoke, 1969; Adeniyi et al., 1970) and that some of the azathioprine-resistant cases may change to a linear pattern of fluorescence (Adeniyi et al., 1970). This pattern of fluorescence is associated with basement membrane antigenicity (Dixon, 1968) and it is possible that azathioprine therapy unmasks underlying basement membrane auto-immunity in these cases. This would mean that the glomerular reaction is biphasic: a stage of immune complex deposition and another of true basement membrane autoimmunity. This possibility may account for the progressive nature of the disease. In this connection Dumonde's finding that masked antigenic determinants may allow autoantibodies to co-exist in vivo with tissue antigens to which they are directed and that in some situations unmasking of tissue antigens may permit access of antibody may be relevant to our situation (Dumonde,

1966) Alternatively soluble complex/basement membrane union may provide a new complex antigen for prolonged immunological activity and account for the persistence of immune complexes as observed by Dixon and others (1961) and also the progression to chronic glomerulonephritis.

Summary

Possible causes of persistence of soluble complexes in Kidney

(1) Size is important as complexes formed in a situation of extreme antigen excess are small and persist for a long time (Weigle, 1964).

(2) With each relapse of parasitaemia complexes appear to persist longer (Ward and Conran, 1969). It is possible that in diseases like quartan malaria where relapses are known to occur over a long period of time persistence of associated soluble complexes occur for considerable periods of time.

(3) Persistence of parasitaemia itself may produce a state of chronic soluble complex circulation. Such a persistence has been shown to occur and to be due to 'parasite variation' in malaria (Brown and Brown, 1965).

(4) The production of low affinity antibodies may be responsible for physical dominance of the antigen though the former may be produced in apparently adequate amounts (Soothill and Steward, 1971). An antigen-excess situation could conceivably persist under these circumstances.

(5) Firm binding of complexes to basement membrane could occur and thus reduce the rate of their removal (Dixon et al., 1961, 1965).

(6) Basement membrane autoimmunity could either be due to masking of antigen determinants thus allowing autoantibodies to co-exist *in vivo* and become active when these are unmasked (Dumonde, 1966) or alternatively this autoimmunity to be secondary to soluble complex deposition (Houba et al., 1971; Kibukamusoke, 1971.)

(7) Tubular damage from immune complex deposition can release modified antigens which could give rise to progressive renal damage as in the case of the self perpetuating nephritis in experimental animals elicited by immunisation with renal tubular antigens (Heymann et al., 1959, Dixon et al., 1968 and Glassock et al., 1968).

Serological changes in malarial nephropathy

Apart from our studies (Kibukamusoke and Voller, 1970) no others are available on changes in immunoglobulins in the nephrotic syndrome of quartan malaria. In these studies a group of 53 cases of the syndrome were studied together with 19 controls.

Table 6.3 shows the results of this study. Four main conclusions can be drawn from this table:

(i) The concentration of serum immunoglobulin-G (IgG) in active cases of malarial nephrosis is slightly lower when compared to that found in controls and cases in full remission. This is most probably due to urinary loss.

(ii) Immunoglobulin-M (IgM) concentration, however, is considerably greater in active cases than in controls and remission cases $(0.05 > P > 0.025)$.

(iii) Malaria antibody titres are significantly higher in active cases than in either controls or remission cases $(0.01 > P > 0.005.)$

(iv) Cases in full remission have titres of malaria antibodies similar to those in controls $(0.10 > P > 0.05)$.

Table 6.3

Serum immunoglobulins and malaria antibody levels in quartan malarial nephrosis

No.	Group	Immunoglobulin levels (mg%)		Malaria antibody levels
		IgG	IgM	
34	Active nephrotic syndrome	$1,572 \pm 163$	467 ± 84	$3,248 \pm 662$
19	Nephrotic syndrome in remission	$1,781 \pm 178$	221 ± 45	$2,852 \pm 801$
19	Controls	$2,392 \pm 165$	230 ± 12	360 ± 144

(From Kibukamusoke and Voller (1970). *Brit. med. J.* **1,** 406.)

Thus it is clear that IgM is the immunoglobulin responsible for the abnormalities in this syndrome. Its increase is accompanied by an elevation in malaria antibody levels. It is therefore possible that the increase is due to malaria antibodies of the macroglobulin type. The disease does not necessarily occur in people with an established immunological abnormality but possibly among those who react with an insufficient antibody response to *P. malariae* antigen, or with low affinity antibodies.

In Chapter 2 emphasis was given to a significant preponderance of people of Rwandan origin in an unselected series and this is the ethnic group whom Shaper (1968) found to have a number of abnormal antibodies in their sera.

Apart from group studies of this kind the situation is not at all clear whether it is the immunologically abnormal person who suffers renal damage from soluble complex disease or whether it is a chance occurrence in the individual who happens to have a slight excess of antigen over antibody during the course of *P. malariae* infection.

The fact that remission cases show the same immunoglobulin-M concentrations as controls suggests that the initial immunological status may not determine the development of malarial nephrosis. However, it is equally possible that the excess of Rwandans in the series quoted above is due to an increased tendency of soluble complex formation occurring among the immunologically abnormal.

That IgM shows such large increases in active cases may mean failure or inefficiency of the switch-off mechanism for IgM formation during the course of infection—and this may be confined to *P. malariae* infection in 'susceptible' individuals. Both IgM and malarial indirect fluorescent antibodies are considerably increased in the nephrotic syndrome and big spleen disease—two diseases thought to be due to abnormal immunological reactions during *P. malariae* infection.

It has been suggested (Sahiar and Schwartz, 1964; Möller and Wigzell, 1965) that termination of IgM synthesis occurring 4–5 days after injection of antigen may be due to IgG synthesis by a feed-back suppression mechanism. IgG starts to appear at this time. This suggestion has been amply confirmed by Britton and Moller (1966, 1968) using a different experimental system. IgG production, however, is dependent on continuous antigenic stimulation (Uhr and Moller, 1968). Regular cyclical fluctuations of cellular IgM synthesis after one antigen injection, e.g. *E. coli* lipopolysaccharide in mice (Britton and Moller, 1968) are probably due to a feed-back suppression of IgM synthesis itself, certain concentrations of IgM antibodies interacting with the antigen in such a way as to suppress its ability to stimulate further IgM synthesis (Britton and Moller, 1968). High IgM concentrations in malarial infections may behave similarly though this may also be due to antigenic variation so ably demonstrated by Brown and Brown (1965). In this case, each antigen variant would stimulate its own IgM antibody. Desowitz *et al.* (1968) working with

Table 6.4

Immunoglobulin levels analysed in relation to malaria antibody titres

	No.	Low malaria antibody levels F.A. titre 320 or less IgM (mg%)	IgG (mg%)	No.	High malaria antibody levels F.A. titre above 320 IgM (mg%)	IgG (mg%)
Active nephrotics	14	223 ± 38	1,354 ± 223	20	638 ± 128	1,763 ± 220
Nephrotics in remission	10	151 ± 22	1,486 ± 266	9	299 ± 88	2,101 ± 234
Controls	14	217 ± 12	2,212 ± 141	5	296 ± 27	3,020 ± 480 (4 values only)

IgG values are almost similar in both groups.
The mean IgM value is much greater in the high malarial antibody group ($0.005 > P > 0.0025$).
(From Kibukamusoke and Voller (1970). *Brit. Med. J.*, **1**, 406.)

P. coatneyi demonstrated a causal relationship between gammaglobulin increase and the course of parasitaemia. They also showed not only an IgG but also an IgM increase.

If the data given in Table 6.3 is re-analysed to show the changes in the given factors in relation to malaria antibody concentration, further information can be obtained (Table 6.4).

It will be seen that the mean IgM value is much greater in the high malarial antibody group (0·005 > P > 0·0025). Thus this change in IgM concentration is directly related to an increase in the titre of malaria antibodies.

If the data are further rearranged in relation to presence of glomerular immune deposits (Table 6.5) it will be found that IgM concentration is significantly higher (0·01 > P > 0·005) when immune deposits are present.

Table 6.5

Serum immunoglobulins and Malaria antibody levels in relation to glomerular immune deposits

Renal immune deposits	No.	Serum immunoglobulins		Serum malaria antibody titres (Reciprocal of F.A. titres)
		IgG (mg%)	IgM (mg%)	
Present	7	1,986 ± 357	523 ± 119	3,763 ± 1,424
Absent	15	1,893 ± 318	241 ± 38	2,587 ± 822

IgM is significantly higher (0·01 > P > 0·005) when immune deposits are present.
IgG and malaria antibody titres are almost similar in both groups. (From Kibukamusoke and Voller (1970). *Brit. med. J.* **1,** 406.)

Thus the immunology of malarial nephropathy is still a challenging problem not only to workers with simian but also to those with human plasmodia. Antigenic analysis of plasmodia (Zuckerman and Ristic, 1968; Zuckerman, 1969) holds promise for the isolation and purification of plasmodial antigens one or more of which may be playing a vital role in the causation of this syndrome. Since plasmodia have been shown to consist of a mosaic of antigens (Spira and Zuckerman, 1966) the task of isolating one in a state of immunologic purity is by no means simple. What is more the offensive antigen may not be a corporal but an exo-antigen.

BIBLIOGRAPHY

Aarons, I. (1964). Renal immunofluorescence in NZB–NZW mice. *Nature*, **203,** 1080.

Adeniyi, A., Hendrickse, R. G. and Houba, V. (1970). Selectivity of proteinuris and response to prednisone or immunosuppressive drugs in children with malarial nephrosis. *Lancet*, **i,** 644.

Allison, A. C., Houba, V., Hendrickse, R. G., de Petris, S., Edington, G. M. and Adeniyi, A. (1969). Immune complexes in the nephrotic syndrome in African children. *Lancet*, **i,** 1232.

Andres, G. A., Seegal, B. C., Hsu, K. C., Rothenberg, M. S. and Chapeau, M. L. (1963). Electron microscopic studies of experimental nephritis with ferritin—conjugated antibody—localization of antigen—antibody complexes in rabbit glomeruli following repeated injections of bovine serum albumin *J. exp. Med.*, **117,** 691.

Becker, E. L. (1953). Molecular weight of antigen—antibody complexes. *J. Immunol.*, **70**, 372.

Boyd, M. F. (1940). Observations on naturally and artificially induced quartan malaria. *Amer. J. trop. Med.*, **20**, 749.

Britton, S. and Möller, G. (1966). In *Genetic Variations in Somatic Cells*, p. 213. Czechslovak Academic Science, Prague.

— (1968). Regulation of antibody synthesis against *Escherichia coli* endotoxin. I. Suppressive effect of endogenously produced and passively transferred antibodies. *J. Immunol.*, **100**, 1326.

Brown, K. N. and Brown, I. N. (1965). Immunity to malaria: antigenic variation in chronic infections of *Plasmodium knowlesi*. *Nature* (Lond.), **208**, 1286.

Cameron, J. S. and Kibukamusoke, J. W. (1971). Plasma C′3 concentrations in malarial nephropathy. *E. Afr. med. J.*, **48**, 466.

Christian, C. L. (1969). Immune-complex disease. *New Engl. J. Med.*, **280**, 878.

Cox, H. W. (1959). A study of relapse *Plasmodium berghei* infections isolated from white mice. *J. Immunol.*, **82**, 209.

— (1966). A factor associated with anaemia and immunity in *Plasmodium knowlesi* infections. *Milit. Med.*, **134**, 10.

Desowitz, R. S., Pavanand, K. and Vacharaphorn (1968). Comparative studies on the pathology and host physiology of malarias. IV. Serum protein alternations in *Plasmodium coatneyi* malaria: a comparison of cellulose acetate and polylamide disc electrophoretic patterns. *Ann. trop. Med. Parasit.*, **62**, 210.

Dixon, F. J. (1962–3). The role of antigen-antibody complexes in disease. *Harvey Lect.*, **58**, 21.

— (1968). The pathogenesis of glomerulonephritis. *Amer. J. Med.*, **44**, 493. (Editorial).

Dixon, F. J., Edgington, T. S. and Lambert, P. H. (1967). Non-glomerular antigen–antibody complex nephritis. In *Immunopathology*. Fifth International Symposium. (Edited by Grabar, P. and Miescher, P. A.) p. 17. Schwabe, Basel.

Dixon, F. J., Feldman, J. D. and Vasquez, J. J. (1961). Experimental glomerulonephritis. The pathogenesis of a laboratory model resembling the spectrum of human glomerulonephritis. *J. exp. Med.*, **113**, 899.

Dixon, F. J., Unanue, E. R. and Watson, J. I. (1965). In *Immunopathology*. Fourth International Symposium. (Edited by Grabar, P. and Miescher, P.) p. 363. Schwabe, Basel.

Dixon, F. J., Vasquez, J. J., Weigle, W. O. and Cochrane, C. G. (1958). Pathogenesis of serum sickness. *Arch. Path.*, **65**, 18.

Dixon, F. J. *et al.* (1968). In *Immunopathology*. Fifth International Symposium. (Edited by Grabar, P. and Miescher, P. A.). Schwabe, Basel.

Dumonde, D. C. (1966). Tissue-specific antigens. *Adv. Immunol.*, **5**, 245.

Eaton, M. D. (1939). Soluble malarial antigen in serum of monkeys infected with *Plasmodium knowlesi*. *J. exp. Med.*, **69**, 517.

Edgington, T. S., Glassock, R. J. and Dixon, F. J. (1968). Autologous immune complex nephritis induced with renal tubular antigen. I. Identification and isolation of the pathogenetic antigen. *J. exp. Med.*, **127**, 555.

Eisen, H. N. and Karush, F. (1949). The interaction of purified antibody with homologons hapten. Antibody valence and binding constant. *J. Amer chem. Soc.*, **71**, 363.

Fennel, R. H., Jr., Pardo, V. and Gibson, L. L. (1965). Experimental glomerulonephritis in rats as related to antigen dosage. *Fed. Proc.*, **24**, 682.

Gilles, H. M. and Hendrickse, R. G. (1963). Nephrosis in Nigerian children; role of *Plasmodium malariae*, and effect of antimalarial treatment. *Brit. med. J.*, **2**, 27.

Gilles, H. M., Lauson, J. B., Sibelas, M., Voller, A. and Allen, N. (1969). Malaria, anaemia, anaemia and pregnancy. *Ann. trop. Med. Parasit.*, **63**, 245.

Glassock, R. J., Edgington, T. S. and Dixon, F. J. (1968). *J. exp. Med.*, **127**, 573.

Greenwood, B. M., Herrick, E. M. and Voller, A. (1970). Suppression of auto-immune disease in NZB and (NZBI NZW) Fl Hybrid mice by infection with malaria. *Nature* (Lond.), **226,** 266.

Greenwood, B. M. and Voller, A. (1970*a*). Suppression of autoimmune disease in New Zealand mice associated with infection with malaria I. (NZBX NZW) Fl Hybrid mice. *Clin. exp. Immunol.*, **7,** 793.

— (1970*b*). Suppression of autoimmune disease in New Zealand mice associated with infection with malaria II. NZB mice. *Clin. exp. Immunol.*, **7,** 805.

Heidelberger, M. and Pedersen, K. O. (1937). Molecular weight of antibodies. *J. exp. Med.*, **63,** 393.

Helyer, B. J. and Howie, J. B. (1963). Renal disease associated with positive lupus erythematosis tests in a cross-bred strain of mice. *Nature* (Lond.), **197,** 197.

Heymann, W., Hackel, D. B., Harwood, S., Wilson, S. G. F. and Hunter, J. L. P. (1959). *Proc. Soc. exp. Biol.* (*N.Y.*), **100,** 660.

Holmes, M. C. and Barnett, F. M. (1963). The natural history of autoimmune disease in NZB mice. A comparison with the pattern of human autoimmune mani-festations. *Ann. Int. Med.*, **59,** 265.

Houba, V. (1971). Personal communication.

Houba, V., Allison, A. C., Hendrickse, R. G., de Petris, S., Edington, G. M. and Adeniyi, A. (1970). In *Proceedings of the International Symposium on Immune Complex Diseases.* (Edited by Bonomo, L. and Turk, J. L.) Carlo Erba Foundation, Milan, Italy.

Houba, V., Allison, A. C., Adeniyi, A. and Houba, J. E. (1971). *Clin. exp. Immunol.*, **8,** 761.

Howie, J. B. and Helyer, B. J. (1965). Autoimmune disease in mice. *Ann. N.Y. Acad. Sci.*, **124,** 167.

Karush, F. (1956). The interaction of purified antibody with optically isomeric haptens. *J. Amer. chem. Soc.*, **78,** 5519.

Kibukamusoke, J. W. (1966*a*). The nephrotic syndrome in Lagos, Nigeria. *W. Afr. med. J.*, **15,** 213.

— (1966*b*). *The nephrotic syndrome in Uganda with special reference to the role of Plasmodium malariae.* M.D. Thesis, University of East Africa, Kampala, Uganda.

— (1967). The examination of multiple slides for the demonstration of malaria para-sites. *J. trop. Med. Hyg.*, **70,** 46.

— (1968). Nephrotic syndrome and chronic renal disease in the tropics. *Brit. med. J.*, **2,** 33.

— (1969). The riddle of malarial nephrosis. *E. Afr. med. J.*, **46,** 12.

— (1971). The nephrotic syndrome of quartan malaria. *Med. J. Aust.*, **1,** 187.

Kibukamusoke, J. W. and Hutt, M. S. R. (1967). Histological features of nephrotic syndrome associated with quartan malaria. *J. clin. Path.*, **20,** 117.

Kibukamusoke, J. W., Hutt, M. S. R. and Wilks, N. E. (1967). The nephrotic syn-drome in Uganda and its association with quartan malaria. *Quart. J. Med.*, **36,** 393.

Kibukamusoke, J. W. and Voller, A. (1970). Serological studies on nephrotic syn-drome of quartan malaria in Uganda. *Brit. med. J.*, **1,** 406.

Kibukamusoke, J. W. and Wilks, N. E. (1965*a*). The appearance of malaria anti-bodies in nephrotic urines. *F. Afr. med. J.*, **42,** 203.

— (1965*b*). Rapid method for urinary protein concentration. Appearance of malaria antibodies in nephrotic urines. *Lancet*, **i,** 301.

Linscott, W. D. and Cochrane, C. G. (1964). Guinea pig beta 1C-globulin: its relationship to the third component of complement and its alteration following interaction immune complexes. *J. Immunol.*, **93,** 972.

McGregor, I. A., Turner, M. W., Williams, K. and Hall, P. (1968). Soluble antigens in the blood of African patients with severe *Plasmodium falciparum* malaria. *Lancet*, **i,** 881.

Moll, F. C. and Hawn, C. V. Z. (1952). Experimental hypersensitivity. Relationship of dosage to serological and pathological responses following injections of heterologous protein. *Proc. Soc. exp. Biol. Med.*, **80,** 77.

Möller, G. and Wigzell, H. (1965). Antibody synthesis at the cellular level. Antibody induced suppression of 19S and 7S antibody response. *J. exp. Med.*, **121,** 969.

Morrack, J. R., Hoch, H. and Johns, R. G. S. (1951). The valency of antibodies. *Brit. J. exp. Path.*, **32,** 212.

Morris, A. and Möller, G. (1968). Regulation of antibody synthesis effect of adoptively transferred antibody producing spleen cells on cellular antibody synthesis. *J. Immunol.*, **101,** 439.

Ngu, J. L. and Monekosso, G. L. (1968). Variation of serum complement levels in the nephrotic syndrome in Lagos, Nigeria. *J. trop. Med. Hyg.*, **71,** 252.

Ogg, C. S., Cameron, J. S. and White, R. H. R. (1968). The C3 component of complement (beta 1C-Globulin) in patients with heavy proteinuria. *Lancet*, **ii,** 78.

Onclay, J. L., Ellenbogen, E., Gitlin, D. and Gurd, F. R. N. (1952). Protein–protein interactions. *J. phys. Chem.*, **56,** 85.

Pappenheimer, A. M., Jr., Lundgren, H. P. and Williams, J. W. (1940). Studies on molecular weight of diptheria toxin, antitoxin and their reaction products. *J. exp. Med.*, **71,** 247.

Rhyne, M. B. and Germuth, F. G., Jr. (1961). The relationship between serum complement activity and the development of allergic lesions in rabbits. *J. exp. Med.*, **114,** 633.

Sahiar, K. and Schwartz, R. S. (1964). Inhibition of 19S antibody synthesis by 7S antibody. *Science*, **145,** 395.

Schwab, L., Moll, F. C., Hall, T., Brean, H., Kark, M., Hawn, C. V. Z. and Janeway, C. A. (1950). Experimental hypersensitivity in rabbit. Effect of inhibition of antibody formation by X-radiation and nitrogen mustard on histologic and serologic sequences, and on behavior of serum complement following single large injection of foreign proteins. *J. exp. Med.*, **91,** 505.

Shaper, A. G. (1968). Immunological studies in a tropical environment. *E. Afr. med. J.*, **45,** 219.

Singer, S. J. and Campbell, D. H. (1951). The valence of precipitating rabbit antibody. *J. Amer. chem. Soc.*, **73,** 3543.

— (1952). Physical-chemical studies of soluble antigen–antibody complexes. I. The valence of precipitating rabbit antibody. *J. Amer. chem. Soc.*, **74,** 1794.

— (1955). Physical-chemical studies of soluble antigen–antibody complexes. V. Thermodynamics of the reaction between ovalbumin and its rabbit antibodies. *J. Amer. chem. Soc.*, **77,** 4851.

Soothill, J. F. (1967). Altered complement component C3A (beta-1C-beta 1A) in patients with glomerulonephritis. *Clin. exp. Immunol.*, **2,** 83.

Soothill, J. F. and Hendrickse, R. G. (1967). Some immunological studies of the nephrotic syndrome in Nigerian children. *Lancet*, **ii,** 629.

Soothill, J. F. and Steward, M. W. (1971). *Clin. exp. Immunol.*, **9,** 193.

Spira, D. and Zuckerman, A. (1966). Recent advances in the antigenic analysis of *Plasmodia. Milit. Med.*, **131,** supplement, 1117.

Turner, M. W. (1967). In *Protides of the Biological Fluids.* Vol. 25, p. 591. Amsterdam.

Uhr, J. W. and Möller, G. (1968). Regulation effect of antibody on the immune response. *Advanc. Immunol.*, **8,** 81.

Unanue, E. R. and Dixon, F. J. (1967a). Experimental allergic glomerulonephritis induced in the rabbit with heterologous renal antigens. *J. exp. Med.*, **125,** 149.

— (1967b). Experimental glomerulonephritis. Immunological events and pathogenetic mechanisms. *Advances in Immunology.* Vol. 6, pp. 1–90. (Edited by Dixon, F. J. and Humphrey, J.). Academic Press, New York.

Voller, A. and Rossan, R. N. (1969). Immunological studies on simian malaria. III. Immunity to challenge and antigenic variation in *Plasmodium knowlesi*. *Trans. roy. Soc. trop. Med. Hyg.*, **63,** 507.

Ward, P. A. and Conran, P. B. (1969). Immunopathology of renal complications in simian malaria and human quartan malaria. *Milit. Med.*, **134,** 10.

Weigle, W. O. (1958). The nature of antigen–antibody complexes formed in rabbits during an immune response to borine serum albumin. *J. exp. Med.*, **107,** 653.

— (1964). Fate and biological action of antigen–antibody complexes. *Advanc. Immunol.*, **1,** 283.

Weigle, W. O. and Dixon, F. J. (1958). Relationship of circulating antigen–antibody complexes, antigen climination, and complement fixation in serum sickness. *Proc. Soc. exp. Biol.* (N.Y.), **99,** 226.

Weigle, W. O. and Maurer, P. H. (1957). The molecular ratios of soluble rabbit antigen–antibody complexes. *J. Immunol.*, **79,** 223.

Wellde, B. T. and Sadun, E. H. (1967). Resistance produced in rats and mice by exposure to irradiated *Plasmodium berghei*. *Exp. Parasit.*, **21,** 310.

West, C. D., Northway, J. D. and Davie, N. C. (1964). Serum levels of beta-1C globulin, a complement component in the nephritides lipoid nephrosis and other conditions. *J. clin. Invest.*, **43,** 1507.

Wilson, R. J. M. and Voller, A. (1970). Malarial S-antigens from man and owl monkey infected with *Plasmodium falciparum*. *Parasitology*, **61,** 461.

Wing, A. J., Kibukamusoke, J. W. and Hutt, M. S. R. (1972). *Quart. J. Med.* (in press).

Zuckerman, A. (1969). Current status of the immunology of malaria and the antigenic analysis of plasmodia. A five-year review. *Bull. Wld. Hlth. Org.*, **40,** 55.

Zuckerman, A. and Ristic, M. (1968). In *Infectious Blood Diseases*. (Edited by Weinman, D. and Ristic, M.) Vol. 1, p. 80. Academic Press, New York.

7 Therapy

It would be expected that a disease due to malaria would respond to antimalarial therapy but if it is realised that the parasite itself plays no part in the actual damage found in the kidneys the lack of response to this form of therapy will be readily understood.

Antimalarial therapy

Experience at Mulago and that of Gilles and his colleague in Nigeria (Gilles and Hendrickse, 1963) and also Houba and others (Houba *et al.*, 1970; 1971), have clearly indicated the non-effectiveness of antimalarial therapy in this syndrome. At Mulago Hospital it was found that the oedema tended to continue building up during antimalarial therapy thus giving an impression of deterioration during antimalarial therapy. This observation is not surprising as one of the important causes of fluid retention in this condition is proteinuria and this continues unabated during antimalarial therapy.

Parasitaemia, which is often scanty, disappears very rapidly on antimalarial therapy (Chapter 3) and workers have consequently recommended that antimalarial drugs should be conscientiously avoided prior to a search of parasites if this is to be successful. The anomalous situation is thus produced where a condition due to malaria progresses for a considerable length of time when the offending parasite has been removed.

Long-term malaria prophylaxis, however, appears to be beneficial and this is most probably due to the prolonged absence of the blood forms of the parasite which are responsible for the production of the offending immune bodies (Kibukamusoke, 1968). Malaria eradication has also achieved the same result (Giglioli, 1962a, b). Camolar (cycloguanil pamoate), a long-acting depot antimalarial, may be used by the intramuscular route in cases where regular prophylaxis is impracticable. These measures are, however, slow in producing the required results either in the individual or in the community and are therefore unwieldy in clinical practice.

Immuno-suppressive therapy

As has already been shown in Chapter 6 the basis of renal damage in quartan malarial nephropathy is immunological. The actual cause of pathological change is the deposition of soluble immune complexes along the capillary basement membrane. It is therefore reasonable to expect clinical response to result from a removal of these immune deposits. This appears to be true of cases who go into a remission whether this be spontaneous or the result of drug administration (Ward and Kibukamusoke, 1969, Adeniyi *et al.*, 1970; Houba *et al.*, 1970 and 1971).

At Mulago some success has been achieved with azathioprine in the management of this syndrome. In 14 such cases in children (Table 7.1)

Table 7.1

Azathioprine therapy

No.	Name	Glomerular histology	Steroid Duration in months	Therapy Result	Results of azathioprine therapy
1	F.S.	Mild prolif.	8	Nil	Complete (8 weeks)
2	Kas.	Minimum focal	5	Nil	Complete (8 weeks)
3	S.K.		5	Nil	Complete (8 weeks)
4	L.W.	Mild focal	24	Nil	Complete (4 weeks)
5	F.K.	Diffuse prolif.	24	Nil	Complete (8 months)
6	S.N.	Mild prolif.	6	Nil	Complete (8 months)
7	Z.S.	Minimum focal	12	Nil	Nil (6 months)
8	Kat.	Minimum focal	12	Nil	Nil (12 months)
9	Mus.	Focal prolif.	2	Nil	Complete (8 months)
10	Rut.	Mild prolif.	2	Nil	Complete (4 months)
11	Obw.	Focal prolif.	1	Nil	Complete (14 weeks)
12	Neet.	—	12	Nil	Complete (8 weeks)
13	J.P.D.	—	24	Nil	Complete (8 weeks)
14	Moh.	Mild prolif.	36	Nil	Complete (8 weeks)

The duration before response to azathioprine is given in parenthasis.
Complete = Total abolition of proteinuria.

a full remission (defined as total abolition of proteinuria) was obtained in no less than 12 cases (Kibukamusoke, 1968).

Further experience at Mulago suggests that the drug requires to be given over a period of many months though in some cases a response can be obtained in as few as two months. In the study quoted above although it was possible to obtain a full remission in eight weeks in some cases, as many as eight months were necessary in some other cases. Subsequent experience has indicated that a beneficial result may require as long as twelve months of therapy. From this experience it is understandable that other workers (Adeniyi *et al.*, 1970) have reported no success in the short periods of their study.

Table 7.2 gives relevant data on 18 other cases in whom a full or a virtually complete remission was achieved.

Figure 7.1 also shows that remission in proteinuria could only be obtained when azathioprine was introduced.

Table 7·2

Clinical data on cases successfully treated with azathioprine

Cases	Age (yr.)	Duration of treatment (in months)	Change in proteinuria	Albumin (g %)	Electrophoresis plasma proteins Beginning/End	Blood urea (mg %) Beginning/End	Cholesterol (mg %)	Renal histology
1	8	7	3+ → Trace	1·2 → 3·5	Slight α_2*	35 → 32	528 → 240	—
2	18	10	3+ → Nil	2·5 → 3·7	Normal*	15 → 18	300 → 133	—
3	7	Irregular 31	3+ → Trace	1·8 → 3·8	Normal*	21 → 27	777 → 172	Minimal change
4	14	15	3+ → 1+	1·9 → 2·7	Normal*	26 → —	205 → 130	—
5	14	3	3+ → 0	2·2 → 3·8	Normal*	6 → 9	210 → 183	Minimal change
6	23	5	4+ → 1+	2·0 → 3·7	α_2B → α_2B	15 → 23	197 → ?	—
7	22	12	3+ → 0	2·6 → 3·4	α_2B → ?	27 → 25	326 → 220	Proliferative with BM change
8	12	7	3+ → 1+	? → 3·5	Normal	22 → 23	354 → 273	Mild proliferative
9	16	4	4+ → 0	1·8 → 4·0	Normal	50 → 18	491 → 183	Minimal change
10	18	4½	3+ → Trace	2·5 → ?	α_2B → Normal	19 → ?	318 → 190	Mild proliferative
11	27	10	3+ → 0	1·2 → 3·6	α_2B → Normal	25 → 17	500 → 168	—
12	15	5	3+ → 1+	2·0 → ?	α_2B → Normal	6 → 7	435 → 280	Mild proliferative
13	5	6	3+ → 1+	1·9 → 2·2	α_2B → Lone α_2	17 → 10	536 → 380	Minimal proliferative
14	40	34	3+ → 0	1·4 → 4·0	α_2B → Normal	14 → 19	391 → 220	Mild proliferative
15	18	8	3+ → 0	1·2 → 3·6	α_2B → Normal	17 → 13	360 → 180	Minimal proliferative
16	10	7	3+ → 0	1·5 → 2·6	α_2B → α_2B	10 → 11	323 → ?	—
17	5	10	3+ → 0	2·5 → 3·7	α_2B → Normal	10 → 20	291 → 190	Mild proliferative
18	14	13	3+ → 0	1·8 → 4·0	α_2B → ?	9 → 8	409 → 208	Mild proliferative

* After treatment.

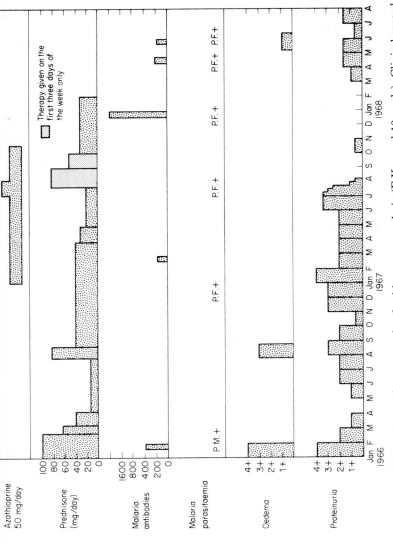

Fig. 7.1. Nephrotic syndrome associated with quartan malaria (F.K., aged 10, male). Clinical record

Azathioprine therapy induced a remission in proteinuria

Re-infection with malaria produced:

(i) an increase of malaria antibodies

(ii) Recurrence of proteinuria ⎱ relapse of nephrotic syndrome

(iii) Appearance of oedema ⎰

It is recommended that a minimum period of 12 months be allowed for azathioprine therapy and it is clear that a special follow-up clinic would be necessary for such patients. Early cessation of azathioprine medication has led to relapses in a large number of initially successful cases. However, if therapy has to be stopped at an early stage then a minimum of eight weeks' therapy *after* disappearance of proteinuria should be observed.

Further work is being done on this problem at the present time.

It is useful to observe strict malaria prophylaxis as this has not only helped to improve general health by providing protection from malaria but also to prevent a return of the immunological events that led to the establishment of the disease. While figures are not available yet on the value of malaria prophylaxis after cessation of azathioprine therapy the clinical impression is that it is useful.

It is logical to expect benefit from post-treatment prophylaxis as not only malaria eradication has led a dramatic reduction in the incidence of the disease (Giglioli, 1962a, b) but prophylaxis has also led to a favourable alteration in the course of the disease (Kibukamusoke, 1968).

To avoid myelosuppression from azathioprine therapy it has been found useful to adopt the use of a small dose such as is used for homograft maintenance therapy: 2–2·5 mg/kg of body weight per day. This dosage schedule has been remarkably free of problems though some have been encountered. Continuation for periods up to two years has therefore been possible without hazard. In fact, a mild leucocytosis is paradoxically observed during the first few weeks of azathioprine therapy at this dosage (Kibukamusoke, 1968).

Improvement of histology has been very difficult to relate to the effects of therapy. Patients with more severe proliferative changes in the glomeruli have shown an improvement towards normal and this has been the experience with workers in West Africa (Adeniyi et al., 1970) but many of those with milder changes do not appear to have achieved a demonstrable improvement in histology. Progression of the lesion, however, appears to have been halted successfully. Proteinuria has been abolished despite persisting mild histological change.

Among the adults azathioprine therapy has led to disappearance of soluble complexes from the glomerular basement membrane (Ward and Kibukamusoke, 1969) and renal function has shown improvement in a number of patients. The events of uraemia and death occurred in 18 per cent of treated as compared with 40 per cent of untreated adult patients with the syndrome. In a few adult cases with minimal glomerular changes a total abolition of proteinuria has been observed (Table 7.2). These experiences are now being examined more critically by controlled studies; but it would seem reasonable at the present time to recommend a trial of azathioprine therapy for the adult patient also.

Hazards of azathioprine therapy

At the dosage used relatively few complications were encountered. A major complication was, however, seen in one case: a child of 5 with a minimum glomerular lesion. This child's lesion was resistant to steroid therapy and she was switched on to 2 mg of azathioprine per kilogram of body weight. After 4 weeks on this dosage proteinuria was gradually diminishing and oedema no longer required diuretic therapy for its control. The child's mother defaulted despite an adequate explanation and easy access to hospital. Four weeks later the child was brought back again in a severe relapse of nephrotic syndrome and therapy was resumed with azathioprine and diuresis. After two weeks on this regimen the child caught a severe pneumococcal pneumonia. She was admitted and given intense treatment with antibiotic combinations and the pneumonia resolved but suppurative peritonitis took its place and the child died a few days later despite intensive treatment. At necropsy the pneumonia was found to have cleared but the peritoneal cavity was full of pus which produced an intense growth of pneumococci. The glomeruli showed minor proliferative change only and the tubules were normal. Death was therefore attributed to pneumococcal peritonitis which must be blamed on azathioprine therapy.

Apart from this patient one adult developed gout in the knees for the first time while on azathioprine therapy. This subsided on withdrawal of the drug. A few children have also developed tonsillitis but as the incidence of tonsillitis was not unduly high it is difficult to ascertain whether immuno-suppressive therapy contributed to its appearance. A number of defaulters who did not have azathioprine for one reason or another also came up with tonsillitis and it is probable that this is merely a reflection of the high incidence of tonsillitis in the community.

Other infections were also infrequently seen. Measles was never seen and cutaneous infections very occasionally. Those who were not on regular malarial prophylaxis did not suffer unduly from malarial fever. Antimalarial drugs are now given routinely at Mulago not for protection against possible undue susceptibility to malaria during immuno-suppressive therapy but for the purpose of suppression of the antigenically active erythrocytic forms.

Azathioprine therapy has, therefore, at this low dosage, been remarkably free of problems particularly among adults. Workers at Mulago are now unwilling to recommend an increase in dosage for the purpose of a possible reduction of the period of therapy as this will necessarily increase the hazards—perhaps a combination of immuno-suppressives might achieve this, but this is not yet known with certainty.

Cyclophosphamide has been tried once (Adeniyi et al., 1970) in this condition when only one of 16 children responded. Further attempts must be made with this drug for periods up to 12 or 24 months before final conclusions can be drawn. This drug, however is not without hazard as in addition to other well recognised toxic effects, azoospermia and ovarian damage may result from its use (Fairley, Barrie and Johnson, 1972).

Steroid therapy

In Europe and North America it has been shown that it is possible to predict those patients who will respond to conventional doses of steroid therapy by studying differential protein clearances (Joachim *et al.*, 1964). Such cases show a highly selective form of proteinuria. If similar studies are performed in an area where malarial nephrosis dominates the practice of nephrology such as Nigeria, the pattern of differential protein clearance is found to be different. Soothill and Hendrickse (1967) and later Adeniyi *et al.* (1970) showed that the poorly selective pattern is frequently seen in children with minimal glomerular change. Steroid responders were found among the few who showed high protein selectivity (Adeniyi *et al.*, 1970). The rate of response in this study was 7 per cent and this rate was similar to that obtained in Uganda (Kibukamusoke *et al.*, 1967).

While studying steroid therapy in this condition Kibukamusoke *et al.* (1967) found that there was better correlation between steroid response and histology. Using very strict criteria for the diagnosis of the 'nil' lesion (*see* Chapter 5) they found that the 'true nil' lesion was very rarely encountered. Criteria for the diagnosis of this lesion included complete absence of even minor local or segmental lesions and the very mild diffuse lesion. These workers found it necessary to count the nuclei in all available glomeruli and diagnosing minimal diffuse endothelial proliferation if such nuclear counts exceeded 120 in any one glomerulus. Small local areas of proliferation may not lead to an increase in the total number of nuclei beyond this level so that it is necessary to search the biopsy specimen for these areas carefully. Only 3 cases with the 'nil' lesion were found in a series of 77 cases (Kibukamusoke and Hutt, 1967) and it was only these three who responded to steroid therapy using the criterion of total abolition of proteinuria for response. It is curious that response was obtained within 10 days of initiation of steroid therapy. It is also considered that these points are directly relevant to the problem of steroid therapy in the nephrotic syndrome of quartan malaria. It is naturally impossible to be sure at the present time whether those patients (showing the 'true nil change') are due to *P. malariae* or not. It may well be that they are representatives of the true lipoid nephrosis of the temperate climates and the high protein selectivity coupled with steroid response (Adeniyi *et al.*, 1970) may be relevant to this. A further point of distinction is that the majority of childhood nephrosis of the temperate zone respond to steroid therapy (Abramowicz *et al.*, 1970) while those who are resistant to them largely respond to cyclophosphamide and not to azathioprine. Malarial cases do not respond to steroids but response has been obtained with azathioprine.

Side effects and complications of steroid therapy

(a) Complications

There were some really alarming complications of steroid therapy though the majority of patients had only minor side effects. Of the severe complications eight were encountered (in over 300 patients):

1. Reactivation of a healed or silent duodenal ulcer occurred in three cases with death from perforation in one patient.
2. Adrenal insufficiency occurred in one child on withdrawal of steroid therapy.
3. Tetany with hypokalaemia in one patient.
4. Hypertension in several patients (fortunately without cerebral or cardiac complications).
5. A severe pneumonia following an apparently simple coryzal illness in one patient (this responded to adequate antibiotic therapy).
6. Pancreatitis in two (with a significant rise in the serum amylase level) and probably a third patient.
7. An acute confusional state in one patient.
8. A spontaneous pneumothorax in one patient.

(b) Side effects

Five side effects were seen:

1. A moon face was invariably present.
2. Acne was seen in a few patients.
3. A scaling dermatosis in 2 patients.
4. Striae in some patients.
5. Hirsuties in one patient.

Diuresis

Oedema is usually severe and ascites is almost always present. Diuresis is therefore required in nearly every patient and it is usually the only form of treatment required in the initial stages of therapy. Among the adults it is often the only reliable form of therapy possible and since oedema is the presenting sign in many cases its effective treatment is imperative.

Oliguria is usual when cases first appear and the initiation of diuresis may be very difficult. The use of relatively large doses of diuretics is therefore recommended in the initial stages and frusemide has been a great help in these patients, particularly adults. Thiazide derivatives are usually insufficient in the initiation of diuresis in the severely affected patients and frusemide has had to be given in doses up to 200 mg twice a day by mouth. However, 80–100 mg orally twice a day are usually sufficient to initiate diuresis but severely oedematous patients with reduced renal plasma flow often need intramuscular frusemide for the first few days. 100 mg given intramuscularly eight to twelve hourly is usually adequate but doses up to 500 mg two or three times a day have occasionally been required. The addition of 50 to 100 mg of oral spironolactone (Aldactone-A) six to eight hourly has helped to initiate diuresis in some of the resistant cases but in others ethacrynic acid (50 mg—8 hourly) has been required in addition.

In still others a plasma expander was necessary in addition to achieve a start of diuresis. Haemaccel (a polymer from degraded gelatine marketed by Behringwerke Ag, West Germany) has been the most effective in our hands. Doses of 50 ml/kilogram of body weight have been used at Mulago in a single dose given intravenously over the course of two hours once a day—and this has needed to be done for two or three days in some patients. Haemaccel has been found useful only if given in addition to the other diuretics as described above and not by itself. Care should be taken, however, as the resulting diuresis may be explosive and lead to severe water and electrolyte depletion. Six litres of fluid were lost over a twenty-four hour period in one case. It is usual to observe a rise in blood urea with the use of plasma expanders but this is usually transient and we have not encountered any major problems from this cause.

Once diuresis is initiated it is relatively easy to maintain it and this may be achieved by the use of a thiazide diuretic in the normal dosage.

Diuretics are usually required for the first four weeks only in children but usually for much longer in adults. However, as the nephrotic state is only a passing phase in this disease it is usual for diuretic therapy to be discontinued after the first few months. Some patients appear never to be able to do without them. The disease is usually severe and rapidly progressive in this group.

Ascites is frequently a problem in adult cases and is usually disproportionate to the degree of oedema especially in the partially treated case. It may thus give an erroneous impression of additional hepatic cirrhosis. Diuresis is sometimes sufficient to deal with the ascites in some patients but paracentesis abdominis may be necessary in others.

Diet

Fluid restriction is often necessary during the initial stages of therapy but frusemide is usually sufficient without this in the later stages. The same is true of salt restriction. It has been possible to maintain many patients on frusemide in an oedema-free state without salt restriction. This has obvious advantages as the patients co-operate more readily with a less restricted and more palatable diet. However, those with significant blood-urea elevation (over 60 mg per cent) are advised to reduce protein intake. It is possible to be more liberal on this in patients whose blood urea is more static. Protein restriction is definitely needed in those with a rapidly rising serum urea level.

Patients on a predominantly vegetable diet, particularly those living on plantains as a staple, maintain their serum potassiums very well even while on heavy doses of diuretics. It is wise, however, to take the precaution of advising a fresh orange or two daily for those on large doses of diuretics.

Hypertension

A large number of adult cases present with hypertension in addition to features of the nephrotic syndrome. In the majority of cases effective reduction of fluid weight is sufficient to control the hypertension though antihypertensive drugs may be required in the initial stages. In a small number of cases antihypertensive drugs are required for long periods and it is then best to employ adrenergic blockers as reserpine has often produced no benefit. The diastolic blood pressure should not be allowed to fall below 100 mmHg if renal failure is present. Patients with reasonably normal renal function (particularly a normal blood-urea level) should have their blood pressures restored to normal levels as far as possible.

Some cases present primarily with renal hypertension or the nephrotic state may recede leaving hypertension as the predominant feature (MacSearraigh et al., 1969). In all these cases control of the blood pressure is necessary as its neglect will add further damage to the kidneys producing a worsening of renal function.

In many patients hypertension settles after some months of antihypertensive therapy but in others treatment is required permanently.

BIBLIOGRAPHY

Abramowicz, M., Arneil, G. C., Barnett, H. L., Barron, B. A., Edelmann, C. M., Gordillo, P. G., Greifer, I., Hallman, N., Kobayashi, O. and Tiddens, H. A. (1970). Controlled trial of azathioprine in children with nephrotic syndrome. *Lancet*, **i**, 959.

Adeniyi, A., Hendrickse, R. G. and Houba, V. (1970). Selectivity of proteinuria and response to prednisolone or immunosuppressive drugs in children with malarial nephrosis. *Lancet*, **i**, 644.

Fairley, K. F., Barrie, J. U. and Johnson, W. (1972). *Lancet*, **i**, 568.

Giglioli, G. (1962a). Malaria and renal disease, with special reference to British Guiana. I. Introduction. *Ann. trop. Med. Parasit.*, **56**, 101.

— (1962b). Malaria and renal disease, with special reference to British Guiana. II. The effect of malaria eradication on the incidence of renal disease in British Guiana. *Ann. trop. Med. Parasit.*, **56**, 225.

Gilles, H. M. and Hendrickse, R. G. (1963). Nephrosis in Nigerian children; role of *Plasmodium malariae*, and effect of antimalarial treatment. *Brit. med. J.*, **2**, 27.

Houba, V., Allison, A. C., Hendrickse, R. G., de Petris, S., Edington, G. M. and Adeniyi, A. (1970). In *Proceedings of the International Symposium on Immune Complex Diseases*. (Edited by Bonomo, L. and Turk, J. L.) Carlo Erba Foundation, Milan, Italy.

Houba, V., Allison, A. C., Adeniyi, A. and Houba, J. E. (1971). *Clin. exp. Immunol.*, **8**, 761.

Joachim, G. R., Cameron, J. S., Schwartz, M. and Becker, E. L. (1964). Selectivity of protein excretion in patients with the nephrotic syndrome. *J. clin. Invest.*, **43**, 2332.

Kibukamusoke, J. W. (1968). Malaria prophylaxis and immunosuppressant therapy in the management of nephrotic syndrome associated with quartan malaria. *Arch. Dis. Childh.*, **43**, 598.

Kibukamusoke, J. W. and Hutt, M. S. R. (1967). Histological features of the nephrotic syndrome associated with quartan malaria. *J. clin. Path.*, **20**, 117.

Kibukamusoke, J. W., Hutt, M. S. R. and Wilks, N. E. (1967). The nephrotic syndrome in Uganda and its association with quartan malaria. *Quart. J. Med.*, **36**, 393.

MacSearraigh, E. T. M., Lewis, M. G., Hutt, M. S. R. and Trussell, R. R. (1969). Renal biopsy studies in Ugandan African women with hypertension in pregnancy. *E. Afr. med. J.*, **46,** 334.

Soothill, J. F. and Hendrickse, R. G. (1967). Some immunological studies of the nephrotic syndrome of Nigerian children. *Lancet*, **ii,** 629.

Ward, P. A. and Kibukamusoke, J. W. (1969). Evidence for soluble immune complexes in the pathogenesis of the glomerulonephritis of quartan malaria. *Lancet*, **i,** 283.

Author Index

Subject Index